# THE

## *Autistic*

# WHOSOEVER

This book is a beautiful read, regardless of your faith, or lack of it. Miya's writing takes us into her world with painful honesty and eloquence. We accompany Miya through her autism diagnosis and her Christian faith, discovering as she did, how both are entwined and how learning over time about what both mean to her, have shaped who she is to today. I read this in one sitting, intrigued to know more. A great book.

*Sarah Hendrickx*
autistic author

With vivid words and a robust sense of humor, Miya Sae paints an informative and inspirational picture of the life of an autistic Christian. It's a treasure to see an individual who's so unapologetic about her faith and her differences. This wonderfully crafted memoir will have readers both giggling over the highly relatable scenarios and wiping away an empathetic tear. Inside these pages is Christianity and neurodivergence at its most pure and base form—no brain-bending theology or head-scratching terminology. It is simply a warm cup of coffee for the soul—mixtures of a bitter past, a flavorful transition, and the warmth of our Savior.

*Moriah Jane*
author and founder of *Finding God in Anime*

This beautifully written, heartfelt memoir allows readers to gain a better understanding of the neurodivergent world, as told through Miya Sae's experiences. Sae is authentically raw, and readers can clearly see God at work through the seasons of her life. *The Autistic Whosoever* will resonate with readers (neurodivergent and neurotypical alike) who may feel alone in their walk to discover how God can use their perceived weaknesses to accomplish His plans.

*Leslie L. McKee*
award-winning author of *Hope Amid the Pain: Hanging on to Positive Expectations When Battling Chronic Pain and Illness*

Miya Sae's memoir of her experience is a story of growth and challenges and a discourse of what one's faith means. She leans into her vulnerability in the hard moments, while deftly weaving in a touch of humor. For anyone who may have felt unseen at any point, this healing journey of embracing life and oneself is for you.

*Judy Liu*
author of *The Vending Portal*

*The Autistic Whosoever* is a wonderfully written, deeply personal journey through the author's life, touching on themes of pain, love, heartbreak, resilience, bravery, self-discovery, and the profound love of Christ. Sae offers powerful insight into what it's like to live with autism, urging us all to advocate for a more inclusive world, where every individual feels seen, valued, and accepted just as they are. God's goodness shines through every page of this soul-stirring story. A beautiful, brilliant read!

*Kathryn M. Inman*
author of *Counting Spoons – a Memoir of Heroin, Heartache, and Hope*

Miya invites us into a sacred place—her hilarious, vulnerable, quirky, and uniquely sweet mind. Miya's ability to color her world and her lifetime of experience and struggle makes her an invaluable voice for us today. She releases us from guilt and shame about our own uniqueness, and into the freedom of God's unconditional love and life with Jesus. *The Autistic Whosoever* is like a delicious, warm, and filling potato dish—and who doesn't like potatoes?

*Bridget Gee*
author of *Single Just Because*

In *The Autistic Whosoever*, Miya Sae demonstrates what autism acceptance and autistic joy can look like as a Christian. She reflects on her successes and struggles, her relationships with family and friends, and how she has deepened her faith in God and her understanding of her autism throughout her life.

Miya is candid about her lifelong search for friendship, fellowship and belonging as an autistic Christian, and her journey to accept God's love while struggling with anxiety, trauma and shame. Her insights challenge the stigma that is too often associated with autism.

This book serves as a powerful source of comfort, reassurance and encouragement for autistic Christians who may be struggling to reconcile their autism with their faith.

*Carolyn Kiel*

host of the Beyond 6 Seconds podcast: Neurodiversity stories from neurodivergent people

AUTISM, CONFUSION,

AND FOLLOWING JESUS

# THE

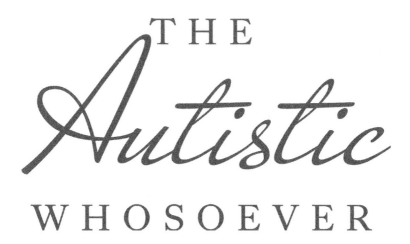

# *Autistic*

# WHOSOEVER

A MEMOIR

# MIYA SAE

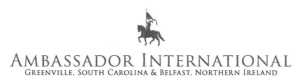

## Ambassador International
### GREENVILLE, SOUTH CAROLINA & BELFAST, NORTHERN IRELAND

www.ambassador-international.com

# The Autistic Whosoever

ISBN: 978-1-64960-892-5, hardcover

ISBN: 978-1-64960-155-1, paperback

eISBN: 978-1-64960-543-6

Cover Design by Hannah Linder Designs

Interior Typesetting by Dentelle Design

Edited by Allison Wells

This work depicts actual events in the life of the author as truthfully as recollection permits. While all persons within are actual individuals, names and identifying characteristics have been changed to respect their privacy.

Unless otherwise marked, Scripture taken from the Holy Bible, New Living Translation, copyright © 1996, 2004, 2015 by Tyndale House Foundation. Used by permission of Tyndale House Publishers, Inc., Carol Stream, Illinois 60188. All rights reserved.

Scripture marked KJV taken from the King James Version of the Bible. Public domain.

Ambassador International titles may be purchased in bulk for education, business, fundraising, or sales promotional use. For information, please email sales@emeraldhouse.com.

AMBASSADOR INTERNATIONAL

Emerald House

411 University Ridge, Suite B14

Greenville, SC 29601

United States

www.ambassador-international.com

AMBASSADOR BOOKS

The Mount

2 Woodstock Link

Belfast, BT6 8DD

Northern Ireland, United Kingdom

www.ambassadormedia.co.uk

*The colophon is a trademark of Ambassador, a Christian publishing company.*

*To the God of my soul. Thank You for the cross. Thank You for wanting to be with me even while seeing the depths of my heart. Thank You for calling out to me that day in 2009 and for all the ways You've worked in and through my life.*

*To my husband. Your love is as close to flawless and unconditional as I've ever experienced from a human being. Thank you for supporting me in all things, even at the highest heights of my anxieties and unpleasantness. I might've never even started this project if it weren't for you.*

*To my faith mentors. Your wisdom is out of this world. Thank you for all the new perspectives you've given me and for being the voices of reason I never knew I needed. Without fail, I always feel a burden lifted after talking with you. You both changed my life and are the kind of women I aspire to be.*

*To my editor, Allison Wells, and the whole team at Ambassador International. Thank you for working with me and taking a chance on me. Thank you for believing in my story.*

*To everyone who alpha read this book, the proposal, and all the other pieces along the way. This book wouldn't be what it is if not for the ways you all challenged me.*

*To all my awesome friends from my angsty teen years until now, who have added so much color to my life. Even though I'm terrible at keeping in touch, I love you all dearly. You know who you are.*

# *Table of Contents*

# Author's Note

Hey, friend. Thanks for stopping by. Regardless of where you are on your journey or whether you're personally autistic or not, the fact that you've picked up this book shows willingness to learn from an autistic person. That's powerful. I'm glad you're here.

With that in mind, I want to give the disclaimer that this book may not be for everyone. There will be moments where I discuss darker things from my past in what I like to call my "B.C. days," or before I was a Christian. While I'm in a much better place now and see things differently than I did then, thanks be to God, I don't want to sugarcoat things. There will be times where I talk about abuse, mention self-harm and suicidal ideation, and, in some chunks of text, roast myself like a turkey on Thanksgiving—sometimes in light-hearted, humorous ways, and other times, not so much. These things may be triggering to some readers or simply not be their cup of tea, which is completely valid. You can put this book down, and I promise we can still be friends.

I will be presenting some ideas and theological views that some may find questionable or unconventional. I don't expect everyone to agree with me. I only ask that you try to keep an open mind while listening to the perspective of someone whose brain works differently from the average person's and whose intentional journey with God has shaped those views. I'm human, and I could absolutely be wrong, but I ask for some grace to be extended. I ask Christian readers to remember that, regardless of differences in theology, we're all siblings on the same path, seeking our Lord together as best as we know how. We may not all be in the same boat, but we're in the same ocean.

To help avoid disappointment, please understand that this is a memoir. It is not a general informational book about autism. There are plenty of excellent books like that out there; and should you ever reach out and ask, I'll happily provide my recommendations. I'm not a professional in this field. I'm just here to give one autistic account through my own experiences.

Note that the names of certain individuals have been changed or withheld and identities kept vague for privacy's sake.

I hope that this story will be useful to you somehow, wherever you're at, even if it's merely a reminder that you're not alone. Thank you for being here.

# Introduction

Hear me out. It's not like I ever actively desired to be an awkward potato. Believe it or not, I didn't wake up one day and ask myself, *What kind of personality should I have? Let's see . . . I know! How about . . . socially inept cringe master, mixed into a batch of intense hyperfixations that people don't care about and topped off with a heaping cup of constant paranoia for good measure? Yeah! Let's do it for the win!*

I mean, I wish I'd had that kind of confidence from the beginning, but it took well over two decades to even start moving in that direction. In the end, the awkward potato life remains, always standing victorious over even the most violent attempts to force it into submission. It's how I came into this world and most likely how I'll leave it. While I take confident ownership of that reality now, it was viewed as unacceptable for most of my life.

Childhood started off rather blissfully. I got to stay cozy at home with my family and cats while coloring, watching cartoons, and above all, feeling safe. Then I was sent into the petrifying world through the fiery gates of school. My identity was confirmed in the years to come because the comments I received were typically of the "Weirdo! Something's wrong with you!" variety. But really, such comments were usually unnecessary efforts in bringing that to my attention. Maybe I had a cool sixth sense that enabled me to pick up on it naturally before anyone said anything. Or maybe it was the fact that nearly every kid I knew ignored me or quite literally ran away from me when I walked by. It could've been either of the two, really.

Trying to blend in or make friends no matter how hard I genuinely tried seemed an impossible feat. I was under the impression that being nice was enough. But as it would turn out, politeness and generally not bothering anyone were still crimes punishable by mockery.

I guess it wouldn't be accurate to say I was always completely aware of my own weirdness. My blissful obliviousness was going strong until the eighth grade, when I somehow caught on and the weight of the situation clobbered me. A revelation rudely pounded on my door: *Oh. So I really* am *an oddball. I've been doing life wrong this whole time.*

Epiphanies are cool and all, but this one left behind unanswered questions and no assistance with my predicament. How do I *stop* doing it wrong? Is there a guidebook or something? Is there a hard reset with a new save file? Some sort of patient and understanding mentor to help me navigate the terrifying world would be ideal.

The author of Hebrews writes, "So we can say with confidence, 'The LORD is my helper, so I will have no fear. What can mere people do to me?'" (Heb. 13:6). Though I wasn't a Christian as a young child, that mentality would've come in handy all those years. I would've felt stronger knowing I had an Ally to take on the formidable opponents of school and social expectations. Where I was standing, each passing day made it pretty clear that I wasn't allowed to go on existing as I was. I needed to figure out how to acquire an entirely new personality if I wanted to be seen with some sort of value and survive among the packs of wolves.

With such a heavy realization hitting me at once like a helicopter dropping bowling balls from the sky and finding that my efforts were futile, I continued asking the universe questions. It was all I knew how to do.

Why am I such a natural loner, and why is that so wrong? How does just saying words to another human lead to fun times and friendship, anyway? How do people always know what to say next like it's a rehearsed movie script? Why am I always saying such cringey, often irrelevant things—that is, if I even manage to speak at all? Why am I so appallingly inept at this giant improv show called life?

Sadly, this is a rather common experience for undiagnosed autistic individuals of all ages. Invisible struggles with no answer or explanation often lead to deep-rooted shame that feels unshakable. In my case, it was usually, "You're just shy, and you need to stop that." Most of the time, we're simply operating in ways that make perfect sense in light of our neurology.

Optimistic teachers thought they would know how to handle me, until I was dropped off on my first day of school and literally bawled nonstop for the entire day straight. What can I say? I didn't understand why I was abandoned like that, left with all those scary strangers in a loud room.

"Don't worry, most kids cry at first. She'll stop soon enough," they said in the morning.

"She . . . hasn't . . . stopped . . . crying," they said at the end of the day.

I don't think I spoke to a single person in school that entire year or in the several years that followed. The crying stopped eventually, which I personally thought was a flex in its own right. Even so, a sizable multitude of concerns from adults would follow as time marched on. Not hanging out with other kids and minding my own business was seen as a critical issue. I couldn't pay attention in class because I was constantly spacing out, thinking about things I actually cared about. Who needs fractions when I could become an anime heroine and fight crime instead?

When the teen years came around, the era of friendlessness and being a shut-in had dragged on so long that my family let me in on the secret: I had something called autism. Finally, an explanation! Except I had no idea what autism was. It just sounded like a fancy medical term that was code for stupid and incompetent, due to it being talked about at home and school as something to be kindly and generously exterminated because everyone needed to be "normal."

Whatever this autism thing was, I was expected to grow out of it with heavy "or else" implications. I was apparently tested at a very young age, though I have no memory of this. The only thing I can recall was being tested as a preteen for something unknown at a psychologist's office. Wires were hooked to my head while I was supposed to do stuff on a computer with my mind. I didn't know what was going on, but it was a free and always welcome pass to skip school. I didn't ask questions. Not having to step foot in the institute of judgment and endless noise was always a blessed relief. I never learned what that test was for or what the results were, but it was apparent to those around me that something was not right about me.

So apparently, I was autistic, though the story kept changing over time.

"What are you talking about? I never said that. You have this other thing, not autism."

"Just kidding, it's this *other* thing."

"*Actually,* you never had anything at all. You were just shy and weird. It's only because you're lazy and selfish, never trying hard enough."

Gaslighting aside, I always had a bit more than a hunch that I was different and not an ideal human. It was always about trying harder and doing better by sheer willpower to act "normal." But of course, trying hard meant nothing unless it produced the desired results. Otherwise, I was lazy and a bad person. Invisible struggles with slower processing time, sensory overload, and executive dysfunction were all written off as some form of insolence. Though I didn't have the first clue about what any of this was at the time or that it was actually pretty normal in terms of neurodivergence, it was evident from a young age that there wouldn't be much grace from the world when I didn't fit the mold.

I would occasionally try to look up what autism was and would always be met with different variations of extremely helpful information. And by "extremely helpful," I mean my findings could be summed up as, "Autism can't really be defined because it looks different in everyone!" In later years, there was at least some information populating in the search. Unfortunately, it was usually a list of dehumanizing stereotypes written in a tone of tragedy, often coupled with the promotion of what many consider to be harmful and traumatizing practices that force autistic people to suppress themselves and pretend to be neurotypical (also known as Applied Behavior Analysis, or ABA), which most autistic people are firmly opposed to. This is one of the many reasons why it's important to learn from autistics themselves. Listen to what we have to say and not what's being said about us.

At long last, I decided to get diagnosed for myself—for real this time. Although it's hard to test for these things in adults, I was officially diagnosed at age twenty-six to be on the "mild" end of the autism spectrum—or what was formerly known as Asperger Syndrome. (I know that most people don't care for terms like "mild" in this context—and I agree and try to avoid it—but that was the diagnosis.) It led to a journey full of delayed lightbulb moments, the more it sank in and the more I learned about autism from trustworthy sources. No more games of "Guess the Ever-Changing Mystery Diagnosis." My level of self-understanding reached new heights, and I was able to finally give myself grace for my unusual behaviors and thought patterns. It was never a case of me not trying hard enough. It's literally how my brain is wired. I'm just a different neurotype—one that I never needed to be sorry for. It's God's design.

It was a long journey getting here. My traits and atypical behaviors were much more obvious during childhood and, by extension, were fought against more aggressively. This is a battle many autistic people face. Reader, if this is you, please know that you're not alone. That type of behavior is, I strongly believe, not how Jesus would treat us if He were here today. He would meet us where we are and delight in us and all of our quirks, regardless of what culture had to say. He would be far more interested in our hearts than the externals.

I want to give the disclaimer that I am *not* an expert on autism nor a mental health professional, and I don't speak for all autistic people. I also know next to nothing about children, autistic or not, so I'm not here to offer parenting advice. Remember that every autistic experience is different. I echo author Sara Gibbs from her excellent memoir *Drama Queen*:

> There will be moments in this book where I draw upon my extensive study and immersion in the autistic community to describe anecdotally common traits or experiences. I in no way wish to claim that these are universal, nor that I speak for all autistic people . . . All I can offer is a tour inside this one autistic brain. Please come in. I'm so sorry about the mess, but there's plenty of comfy seating.[1]

I am simply here to share my own experiences and offer some perspectives. In certain ways, this won't be a super regular memoir. Some parts are my backstory, and others are just straight info-dumps about things I've learned and views I hold. It's my hope that the whole variety can provide insight.

Note that whenever I use the term "neurodivergent," I'm usually referring to autism; however, it can also include ADHD, OCD, dyslexia, Tourette's Syndrome, or any other neurology that isn't considered to be the norm by larger society. "Neurotypical," on the other hand, is pretty much what it sounds like—people with what's considered typical brain wiring who aren't neurologically disabled. "Allistic" refers to someone who isn't specifically autistic but not necessarily neurotypical.

I've found that, in terms of language, the majority of the community prefers "autistic" as opposed to "has autism." For that reason, I try to stick with the former as much as possible, though when it comes to how I'm addressed personally, I'm fine with either. The only thing I find upsetting is when people (especially allistics) try to police us, forcefully telling us what terminology we are and are not allowed to use when describing ourselves and our own experiences. In the disability community, this kind of behavior is referred to as "able-splaining" and should be refrained from being used. When in doubt, it's always good to ask someone what they prefer.

Prior to becoming a Christian, I deeply despised myself and the world. There will be moments when I discuss this because the reality is that autistic people are commonly taught to hate themselves by peers and society. Those parts, among others, may be less-than-comfy to read, but I want to paint an accurate picture in this raw account of an autistic experience.

I remember my mind shattering in utter astonishment a few years ago, the first time I heard someone say that autism is a good thing that doesn't necessarily need a cure. All my life, I heard autism was a tragic disease that needed to be destroyed, end of story. It never occurred to me that it can be a beautiful and valuable thing that uniquely makes us who we are. I never imagined it possible that I'm valid just the way I am, quirks and all, and that I'm not a broken or defective toy that should've been returned for a refund.

The way it was talked about in my younger years, autism also sounded like something only children have and that they would grow out of it eventually. A lot of people still believe this—like my past self did for far too long—but let's bust that myth right now because it's absolutely false. Many of us have simply mastered the art of masking—suppressing visible autistic traits in order to appear neurotypical.

In this day and age, we have more access to information and resources than ever before, yet autistic people are still gravely misunderstood. We often get left out of the diversity and inclusion agendas. Professional settings are open to promoting equality and having neurodivergent people on their teams, until it becomes inconvenient or uncomfortable. We often get placed in boxes because so much of society's supposed understanding is based on stereotypes. Things like executive dysfunction and sensory overwhelm get confused with laziness and entitlement. Our different ways of processing information and interacting with others are perceived as rudeness and low intelligence. In church culture, our traits that make us different get labeled as sinful.

This needs to be talked about more. The heart of the conversation is found in our stories. I'm here to offer mine.

All the messy pieces of my life have come together as this: I am a follower of Jesus Christ, unashamed of the autistic brain I was given. I want to use this book as an opportunity to be a voice, small as it may be, and hopefully reach my fellow, misunderstood autistic adults and offer encouragement. I'm here to tell the story of why I chose to follow Jesus in the first place, how autism has impacted my journey, and how I came to accept my own brain as a Christian who lives and thinks differently from the average person.

Welcome to my silly world.

# PART ONE

## Why I Became a Christian

11

# CHAPTER ONE
## A Swell Beginning

The first time I died, I was furious. On the bright side, the location of my untimely death was quite beautiful. The scene was set with bright skies dotted with small, fluffy clouds; soft green grass beneath my feet as I ran; palm trees galore; and a shimmering lake behind me with the fresh sound of serene waterfalls. It was a five-year-old's paradise. That is, until I lost everything—all because of some wretched crabs and spikes. But after I lifelessly plummeted down to the depths of the island, I was revived and sent back to the beginning, only with empty pockets. Of course, I'm referring to a fictional death on the original *Sonic the Hedgehog* game.

Despite the temporary moment of rage and shaking my fist at the TV, all was well. I was smiles and sunshine again moments later. I turned to my cousin Matt—my best friend, partner in crime, and ultimate role model—basically the older brother I never had, even though we were the same age. We cackled in unison as I handed the controller back to him, figuring it was more fun to simply watch him play because he was objectively the coolest person in the world.

After this typical gaming session of ours, we proceeded to engage in our other go-to activities: riding scooters all over the place, playing makeshift basketball games, and digging through the desert mountain in my backyard looking for "fossils" that would definitely make us rich. We traded cards, watched movies, and feasted on our favorite junk food. Life was good, even when we returned for another night of gaming and I died—again.

Little did I know that this type of metaphorical death wouldn't be the only one I'd experience. In just shy of a decade, I would experience a new kind of death—one by which I wouldn't have to be sent back to the beginning and left to fend for myself. It would be a death to myself and surrender to the God Who gifted me this nice little life in the first place.

But telling that to a kid who was still learning how speak in complete sentences would probably just freak her out. Plus, that would take the fun out of it. No one buys a game only to watch a video of the ending scene, rather than playing through it and experiencing the adventure.

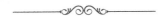

Before I get ahead of myself, let's start with the basics. Usually, the initial question in regards to my faith is whether or not I was raised Christian. My best answer is *kind of.* I obeyed the small handful of loose routines but certainly wasn't a Christ-follower.

Before dinner each night, my family would recite the following prayer: "We thank You, God, for this food. In Jesus' name, amen."

This generic routine was usually followed by my silent, "Okay, whatever, let's eat now." When I was young, we went to a nice Lutheran church on Sunday mornings. Songs were played, and pretty candles were lit. My grandparents on both sides were actively involved in church, and it was a special time for all of us to go hear the Word.

I hated every minute of it. Of course, I wasn't allowed to say that. All church meant to me was having to spend an excruciatingly boring couple of hours sitting still in a relatively dark room while some old guy rambled about things I didn't understand and listening to people play weird music while everyone looked stiff. I felt like I was crammed into a pickle jar, desperate to be released from its confines into the open air. Sitting still and being quiet were natural for me but only on my own terms. Remaining outwardly polite, I'd zone out and desperately hope I wouldn't be asked what I thought of service afterward, since I was too busy imagining what kind of superhero I'd be while trying not to fidget or breathe too loudly.

Sunday school was out of the question, given my difficulties around unfamiliar humans. I probably would've been worse off than simply being bored in service. At least that was safe.

Needless to say, I didn't comprehend anything and had next to no knowledge about God, despite the exposure to that environment. I didn't even understand Jesus and what He was all about—just that I heard His name occasionally and that He was supposed to be important or something. I never even watched *Veggie Tales*. That's how you know I was clueless about this whole Christianity thing.

But I was fine with tolerating church, since it was only on Sundays for an hour. Once free, I'd gleefully return to my hyperfixations at home, while snuggling with my cats and breathing easy in my cozy room decked out in nerdy fandom merchandise. We were privileged to live in a grandiose, newly built house on a mountain, with plenty of space for young kids to frolic and have all kinds of creative fun. From pool parties to building forts to water balloon fights to rock collecting, there was rarely a dull moment.

That's not to say that onlookers never found my hobbies to be dull, but I was perfectly content. While I enjoyed those active things, the large majority of my time was spent gaming and watching my favorite shows. Both would give me jolts of euphoria that sent me to the top of the world, while continuously learning about life through story and imagery. I'd carry that dose of adrenaline with me as I went out to ride bikes with my siblings and cousins or while jumping from the stairs onto generously sized pillows we'd pull from the couch. As long as I could spend a sufficient amount of time engaging in my passions, everything was an adventure. I was on cloud nine with my energized brain.

One of my favorite things was riding my scooter down the concrete slope attached to our driveway. It was always the best during winter when the temperature wasn't comparable to the scorching gust that assaults your face when you open the oven. The exhilaration from the speed, the gentle breeze through my hair, basking in the—

*Clonk!*

That was the sound of my wheel hitting a pebble, effectively sending me flying onto the pavement.

As I cried out in agony, my parents comforted me and patched me up. I got a snack, and all was well with the world again. They tucked me into bed that night and told me they loved me, as per usual. I rested easy, feeling safe in that assurance, even while knowing I had to go to school the next day.

School was by far my greatest source of distress, with all the social expectations and sensory overwhelm, but that was okay because at least I had a good home life. I knew that my family members were the constants in my life and that their personalities would never change. Right?

# CHAPTER TWO
## *Lovingly Hateful Kinship*

"Hello? Is anyone home? Someone let us in! It's hot out here!"

"Why aren't you waking up? *Hello?*"

Coming home from school one day to find one of my guardians passed out on the couch, overdosed, wasn't something I was prepared for at ten years old.

My sibling and I were locked out of the house for hours, relentlessly pounding on the door and ringing the bell. We weren't allowed to have cell phones or house keys yet. Our only option was to sit out there in the agonizing Phoenix heat and wait.

After an eternity, the door opened, and behind it stood our youngest sibling—a mere toddler who had somehow figured out how to reach the lock. We all assumed our family member was just extremely tired, like usual, so we went on with our day and watched cartoons, not thinking much of it until the next morning.

Said family member thankfully survived, but our lives were still about to be snatched up and pummeled by dramatic changes and shattered images.

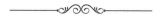

I thought the days when my family all loved each other and every adult was a role model to be looked up to would last forever. There's an old family photo from one of our many large gatherings. Everyone is happy and smiling pretty. I'm six years old, holding Jordan, my stuffed bunny. Matt is standing next to me. He and I had recently discovered an awesome new computer game, which we had to pause to come outside for the picture. While we played, all of the adults were in the other room, talking and laughing and being merry. Our family was safe and wonderful.

When I turned ten, the glass of the frame cracked. With divorce on the horizon, I watched as the narrative around nearly every family member flipped—like a vicious hailstorm knocking fragile cherry blossoms from their branches, bringing the petals of former perceptions to the ground to be trampled. Everyone was actually crazy. They should all be put in prison, depending on whom you asked. Hearing about their latest court cases eventually became mundane, though I was expected to choose the correct side and hate the opposing party. My life shifted into a series of one-sided correspondences that resembled the following:

"That person doesn't even care about you! How can you still love them? They'll leave you to die!"

"Tell (insert name here) this script I'm giving you. If they lash out, just get over it. What *I* want is what *you* want. Understand?"

"If you ever talk to that person again, that's the worst possible thing you could ever do to *me*."

"Be sure to keep the doors and windows locked at all times. You never know if violent so-and-so will come after you out of spite toward me."

One moment, I was enjoying a festive family gathering, wishing it would never end. The next, I was hiding in my bathroom from some of those same people and calling the police.

The very dramatic (first) divorce was final when I was twelve. Then came a complicated split-custody schedule, followed by an endless game of, "We would *never* put you kids in the middle—except we're going to do exactly that every chance we get."

We all went to counseling for a of couple years during the divorce process, which was a great idea in theory, though I didn't really understand why we were being forced to meet with some random guy we didn't know. I did not want to spend my limited free time after school talking to Dr. Ed. That was my time to engage in my hobbies and unwind before I had to go back into sensory survival mode the next day.

Even though the whole thing felt like a waste of time and Dr. Ed had an infantilizing tone that ticked me off, I eventually started opening up about the family dysfunction. That's when things got exciting.

"Miya! You are one of the most negative people I've ever met!" Dr. Ed enthusiastically proclaimed.

The drama would go away if I just changed my attitude and stopped complaining. My takeaway was that either this guy was fully committed to not taking me seriously or everything was mostly, if not all, my fault. Regardless, I held onto hope that things would settle down and be all right in the end. In the meantime, my comforting activities of interest were always waiting for me at home.

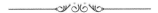

If I'd had a genie as a kid, I would've wished for Matt to move in with us. Riches and superpowers sounded cool and all, but this was far more important. If he were to be my adopted brother, I'd have a friend and would never feel alone again. Of course, he would probably make other friends if that happened, while I remained a loner and got left behind—but that possibility never crossed my mind. Thanks to my autistic trait of mimicking, I went to great lengths to act like him whenever I was around other people. I made sure I spoke the exact same way by drawing from my brain's chaotic notebook of "Matt quotes" and rehearsing in private, all while hoping that others would view me with the same fondness I had for him. Sadly, my copycat attempts did not measure up to O.G. Matt's awesomeness. All that hard work was for nothing.

He liked wrestling, so I liked wrestling. He liked football, so I tried very hard to pretend to like football. The first time I tried eating dry ramen, I thought it was just a notch above inedible. I later found out that dry ramen was Matt's favorite snack. I liked dry ramen after that. Matt was my role model, and I thought I could conquer life if I was just like him. I may not have had friends, but I always had my cousin—*had* being the key word.

Throughout all the madness of this soap opera of a divorce, we drifted from other relatives as well. Before I knew it, Matt felt like a stranger to me. Growing up made us too different, no longer able to enjoy the same things or interact in any way that wasn't forced. I lost my partner in crime, and I was salty.

There seemed to be a tension between the whole family that wasn't there before; or if it was, it wasn't this obvious and heavy. It was bizarre having to change my view of family members as I was being instructed and heartbreaking that we couldn't keep it together after all the happy times of old. No one could be trusted anymore, except for the *definitely* good guys— unless they stepped out of line.

This was particularly earth-shattering as an autistic kid, as many of us tend to be very trusting. All the uprooting of no-longer-trustworthy individuals made for an amplified sense of both confusion and betrayal. But that was supposed to be okay because the Still-Good Guys who were doing the slandering and would absolutely never betray me could always be depended on. Just take their word for it and don't question it.

The more convincing the argument, the more I sided with that person. And sadly, a lot of it was legitimate. Things like unapologetic substance abuse, petty conspiracies, and painfully obvious lies don't exactly help one's case. Those flashy things conveniently distracted from the more subtle issues that would manifest years later.

As an autistic rule-follower, I did as I was told and kept busy with my fun little distractions. I went with the flow, being taught never to argue with authority, *or else.* Of course, that changed whenever one authority figure told me to argue with another one. I began to learn that the world was far less black and white than I'd thought.

For better or worse, I was stuck in my own head most of the time. Whether it was rewatching the same episodes of my favorite shows forty thousand times as a comforting routine, playing the same video games for hours on end, or becoming sort of attached to inanimate objects, I was off doing my own thing and enjoying life in the ways I could. I voluntarily slept on a cot in my room so that my stuffed animals could have the bed. They deserved to be comfortable. I was a very good caretaker of them because that was the rule if I wanted them to come to life and hang out with me. I'm sure it wouldn't freak me out at all if my dragon plush suddenly started flapping around.

It was a weird time of being lonely and not realizing it; being physically surrounded by people most of the time but still feeling alone. Fictional fantasies in my head kept me going. It was a world where I could make life awesome and keep it that way. Plus, I was busy on a mission to never act like a girl.

Growing up around a lot of boys my age, I wanted to fit in and essentially be one myself. Girls were the so-called weaker version of the human species in every way, according to my young male peers, so I obviously didn't want to be one of those. I pretended to like sports, even though I couldn't care less about them. I tried to force myself to like rap music, especially the heavily explicit stuff, much to my parents' horror. I tried to get into wrestling and violence in general because that all seemed to be cool and what all the "bros" were into. I went an embarrassing number of years claiming that mushy things like love and affection were "girly" and that I was above them—whatever that was supposed to mean. I dressed in boys' clothing often because I hardly felt like one of the guys when I was wearing skirts.

All this effort was made, only to find out later that I was absolutely not fitting in with these males I looked up to and nobody bought the act. I've never been a very good faker. But I totally thought I was edgy.

Years later, something life-changing happened: the movie *Aquamarine* was released. I became a mega fanatic, watching it multiple times a day like my life depended on it. I didn't actually care about the whole mermaid thing but, rather, was intrigued by the two main human girls. This was the turning point that sparked the desire to be more feminine—not that I really knew how or what it even meant beyond stereotypes. I wanted to be like the girls in that movie, thinking it would shed my perceived weirdness. At one point, I tried to dye my hair with aquamarine highlights like JoJo's character had, only to be disappointed that they came out puke green instead.

Take two: obtain teal highlight clip-ins and see how long the kids at school believed it. Maybe people would notice me if I had cool hair. And it worked! Then my fifteen minutes of middle school fame passed.

On top of the fact that those clip-ins were straight and glossy while the rest of my hair was a hot mess of greasy waves akin to that of a washed-up sea witch, a girl started messing with it and saw the white plastic at the top.

"It's a clip! Everyone, it's a *clip!* She lied!"

Mission failed. But I supposed the small amount of positive attention I got was nice while it lasted.

In this very awkward phase of preteen life, my thoughts could be summed up as, *I need to change every last thing about me immediately. This is an emergency mission!*

All the while, the loud drama at home lived on. More people were being added to the "Do Not Trust" list—not to mention the continual reminders that any day, I could be abducted or murdered by people who were once safe and dependable. I ultimately concluded that everything was a rose-colored lie. Everything is conditional. Nothing is permanent. People change their minds all the time.

Even so, I somehow didn't fall into complete despair in the midst of this. The God I didn't yet know kept the smoldering wick of hope alive somewhere deep within. As a passage I later came to favor goes, "He will not crush the weakest reed or put out a flickering candle. He will bring justice to all who have been wronged" (Isa. 42:3).

# CHAPTER THREE
## I'm Not a Chatterbox or Australian

Picture this: it's 2007. You're walking into class as an angsty middle schooler, where you're required to be cool and only associate with other cool people. You see that one kid sitting alone, sporting the look of borderline obesity, eyebrows that are half-shaved off, excessive acne adorning a face that looks like it was dunked in oil, greasy hair that snows dandruff like it's the North Pole, and clothing like that of a confused hippie. She's aggressively biting and picking at her nails, pouting, and frequently staring at people but rarely ever talks. Whenever she does speak up at inexplicable moments, it's always a cringe party—which is saying a lot, considering it was middle school.

Now try and guess how many other thirteen-year-olds wanted to be friends with her. Back then, you were already disqualified from being cool if you weren't at least wearing trendy brands. I couldn't even meet that minimum requirement. It was all too tight and too pricey, and I was far too edgy for that stuff. Combine the illegal tween fashion choices with all my quirks and crown me the winner of the hot mess tournament—should there ever be one. But I didn't know this. I was ready to rock the oversized hotel receptionist shirts until the day I died.

Before the awkward middle school days, I never thought about my social standing. I'm sure that was for the best, as it made life easier and I didn't hate myself so much. I was content in just vibing and being my oblivious, unashamed self. Spending my time doing the things I loved made me feel alive, even if I was a loner. But there came a time when the reality of the situation was no longer something I could ignore. I couldn't keep disregarding people's perceptions of me or the lonely "other-ness" I was experiencing. It turned into an all-consuming obsession, for which I needed a game plan.

"Maybe if I was skinny, I would suddenly be liked by all," I said aloud to myself.

"Brilliant!" I responded. "Okay, I'm gonna lose weight."

*Nope, I'm still an awkward human.*

"'Kay, so that didn't really work. Maybe it wasn't enough. Don't sweat it, self. Let's try makeup and maybe smiling more."

*Negative.*

"Well, maybe if I was more social and didn't say stupid things all the time?"

My optimistic half gave up. "But how? How do people do this? What am I even supposed to talk about? How do I immediately know what to say when people go off the script?"

Everyone made it look so easy. From where I was standing, it felt like trying to knit an intricate sweater while bungee jumping.

Contrary to popular belief, the seemingly simple act of communicating with other humans doesn't come naturally to everyone—namely, neurodivergents. Even if someone is physically able to speak, that doesn't necessarily mean their brain tells them to or gives them words all the time. It can be particularly overwhelming in a culture where we're all expected to be quick-witted and have a never-ending supply of appropriate responses immediately ready to hand out in any given situation, while also making sure to find an adequate time slot to speak without interrupting or getting spoken over. All the while, we have to maintain the "correct" tone of voice, facial expressions, and body language in every subtle form.

There was a silver lining, though. I technically could talk to people all day, as long as it was a topic I wanted to discuss. And by "discuss," I mean talk *at* you in a session of incessant info-dumping about my obsession of the moment. Naturally, people didn't tend to go for that, so I lived in my head. But I very much enjoyed being a "space case." Why waste energy talking to people when I'm already having fun inside my mind? I've always had the common autistic tendency of hyperfixating on things I'm interested in, whether it's my favorite show or video game, a particular band or musician, or a character I made up and inserted into a fictional world. If I'm not partaking in the thing, I'm daydreaming about the thing. In neurodiversity, we call these passionate fixations "special interests."

I couldn't stop fervently fantasizing about fictional characters, no matter how hard I tried or no matter how many adults told me to snap out of it. It's not like there's a switch that I can simply turn off, as convenient as that would be. I later learned that this is often referred to as "maladaptive daydreaming," though I don't typically use that term anymore because I don't like the negative connotations. In my case, it wasn't always to escape from reality during hard times. It was just something that was fun and natural for me. Like breathing. What do other people think about in their free time, anyway?

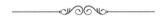

"Are you British? No? What about Australian? Not that either? Are you sure? Then . . . Irish? You definitely have an accent, in case you didn't know."

These are questions you'll probably ask when you hear me speak for the first time. You'll wonder what my strange accent is and why it seemingly comes and goes. If I had a dollar for every time I was asked these things, I'd be able to afford surgery that could potentially fix the problem.

In other words, no, I don't have an accent. There was nothing in my life that could've caused one. I'm from a desert town in Arizona, and no one who raised me had accents. There's no cool backstory of where I came from.

The reality is rather anticlimactic. I have a mild speech impediment, or rhotacism, where I'm physically unable to pronounce the letter "R" most of the time. That's it. I don't know why, but that's how it is and how it's always been. Speech therapy couldn't fix it. There's nothing I can do about it.

In the past, I'd often just say, "Yeah, that's right. I'm from Boston. I'm from England. I'm from Australia. Whatever you say, man"—all while desperately hoping that they wouldn't ask questions about those places, since I knew nothing. It was still easier than having to explain my situation, especially given the fact that most people didn't really care and were just trying to make small talk—or be condescending, in some cases. The unfortunate reality is that having a speech impediment comes with a lot of stigma and is often attributed to a lack of intelligence. It seems to give people the idea that I'm incompetent and can't be taken seriously.

A typical interaction usually resembles the following: "No, 'R' as in 'rabbit.' No, not 'wabbit.' No, not 'labbit.' *Rabbit.* You know what, just give me a pen and paper. No, not 'papuh.' No . . . "

But it is what it is. Overall, I've gotten to a place where I've mostly accepted it and have gotten better at speaking as a whole with time. These days, I say my impairment is a feature, not a bug.

Growing up with crippled speech, however—that's another story. It was kind of hard to be a cool, edgy teen when I was constantly handing out free ammunition to mock me to everyone within hearing range. This was part of the reason why I didn't talk much as a kid, on top of the fact that the idea of conversing with others didn't register in my brain half the time. Why was I supposed to talk to the other kids when I didn't feel like it and didn't know them?

Quietness became less acceptable as I aged. I had been on metaphorical crutches my whole life, surviving in the shadows, only to be suddenly shoved onto a track in front of an audience and told to run ten miles. It's what everyone was "supposed" to do, so no excuses and no complaining. Just get up and do it—the same way as everyone else.

This kind of thing wasn't unique to just me. Such expectations are woven into the fabric of society, providing extra, unreasonable challenges to neurodivergent people who can't pick them up instinctively like their neurotypical peers and need a good deal of support.

The daily marathon running of tween social expectations was an added terror to my biggest nemesis: publicly speaking to a caged audience—probably better known as class presentations. I would've been mostly fine with the planet bursting into flames before I had to walk up there and force everyone to listen to my pain-inducing garbage, enhanced by shaky hands, voice cracks, and clumsy hair twirls every three seconds. Eye contact? That's funny. I knew how harshly I'd be judged and that I'd likely be penalized for not speaking clearly, thanks to the speech impediment. The frustrating reality that the volume of my voice can't go very high didn't help matters.

For years, I'd find time to hide away and practice pronunciation. Everything would sound fine to my own ears when I spoke out loud, and I was at a loss as to what everyone was complaining about. Then I'd hear a recording of my voice. I wanted to shrivel up and die. I sounded like a five-year-old who had just been punched in the gut and was trying not to cry. That was all the more reason to remain the quiet kid.

Even before becoming aware of this speech dilemma, I just wouldn't talk to people, other than family and people who came over often. This wasn't out of any kind of stubbornness; it was simply my natural default. There were those rare occasions when someone would come up and try to talk to me and I would stare at them, ignore them, or walk away completely. I legitimately didn't see anything wrong with that for a long time. But apparently, it's considered impolite to completely disregard people when they're speaking to you.

This kind of behavior is commonly labeled as selective mutism, or the inability to speak in certain situations due to extreme social anxiety. That was one of my many ever-changing diagnosis stories. There was probably a shade of it as a comorbidity at the time, but I wasn't all that anxious yet. Ironically enough, most of the social nerves activated later on when I *did* start talking at school and realized that I was apparently doing it wrong and couldn't say the right things or read unspoken cues and act accordingly.

It would basically play out like this: "Come on, Miya! Speak up! Be louder and talk more! Er . . . No, not like that."

Before the crashing and burning that began in the tween years, I simply didn't speak in public settings because it felt unnatural. I was in my zone and perfectly content there. The unspoken requirement (pun fully intended) of talking to everyone in range was supposed to be a given, but I didn't pick up on it. I was fine in my bubble and had nothing to say to those people.

It seemed like everyone else was always getting in trouble with the teachers for being too loud or talking too much. I figured if I didn't talk, I'd stay out of said trouble. That logic unfortunately didn't get me too far, since it seemed I was still always getting yelled at everywhere I went. That always scared the living daylights out of me. It's common for autistic people to not like loud noises. For me, the worst sound is yelling. That's where the real mutism gets triggered. If you want a surefire way of making me freeze up and be unable to think, raise your voice at me. (Please don't.)

I didn't understand why I was on the receiving end of these one-sided screaming matches most of the time. The assumption was that I was supposed to just intuitively "get it," but I simply saw it as a part of life, like an afternoon game of golf that adults enjoyed as a hobby.

---

"Is your name Maya?"

"No, it's pronounced MEE-yuh."

"Cool. Maya. Got it."

It was kind of interesting, being simultaneously invisible yet visible enough for a few people to identify me as an easy target for inevitable bullying. Having a name that no one could pronounce didn't help.

The flashiest hater in middle school was a kid named Donald, who was repulsed by my existence for some reason and would always go out of his way whenever he saw me to say nasty things in a dramatic fashion. I'd never met this kid. My nickname became "the crazy woman," and I wasn't allowed to forget it. There was Casey, who took delight in always pointing out that I had no friends. I'd sometimes cross paths with Jen, who was my friend at one point by some miracle but phased me out because I was embarrassing and she was not a fan of my love language of relentless info-dumping about video games. Then there were random people who enjoyed quoting dumb things I'd said in the past.

School was a game of dissociating during the constant loud chatter and chaotic crowds, combined with trying to survive the semi-regular schedule of hostility without snapping and assaulting the offenders. But all things considered and compared to horror stories I've heard from other autistic people, I do think I got by relatively unscathed. I was lucky in that way. Though it had its own harmful effects, I was more invisible than anything most of the time.

Overall, the kids like Donald and Casey who did say things simply weren't afraid of pointing out in their own ways the weirdness they perceived. In time, any remaining naivety took off running and left me alone with my questions on what to do about it.

It was always such a wonder why no one else sat alone at lunch or covered their ears when stepping into the loud cafeteria. I couldn't understand why people always went out on the weekends to socialize instead of staying home in their rooms, where it's safe and a constant performance isn't required. Even more so, how everyone else had so many friends who didn't get sick of them was far beyond me.

I concluded that it wasn't just those kids who were bold enough to be vocal about it who thought I was an insufferable embarrassment to the human race. Probably every living and breathing human in existence was silently judging me every waking moment, as if no one had anything better to think about than me and my oddball personality.

The internal whispers kept growing louder, quickly turning into an obsession: *Stop being the way you are. It's embarrassing. Quit being stupid already!*

*Hit yourself in the head repeatedly, and maybe you'll knock some of the stupid out of there. Just kidding, you're hopeless. But* ha! *I can't believe you actually hit yourself! Talk more! What's wrong with you? Are you* trying *to remain an outcast? But also don't talk because you have nothing good to say, your speech impediment sounds ridiculous, and your voice sounds like that of a little boy who's been gargling nails. No one wants to listen to that.*

In reality, it's likely that very few people were actually thinking about me at all. That's what often happens when I give power to the whispered demonic lies—I become a paranoid mess, obsessing to the point of resenting people before they'd even said or done anything and being fully convinced of things I literally made up.

My life could be summarized as existing in a strange contradiction of being both oblivious to my weirdness and painfully aware of it at the same time. But once it was in my head, I couldn't go on acting like my social standing wasn't a blazing trash fire. My twisted mindset fixated on this, and I started to believe that appearances and reputation were the most important things in the universe. Jesus once called religious leaders with that type of attitude "'whitewashed tombs—beautiful on the outside but filled on the inside with dead people's bones and all sorts of impurity. Outwardly you look like righteous people, but inwardly your hearts are filled with hypocrisy and lawlessness'" (Matt. 23:27-28). In a non-religious way, I had that sort of vision for myself and the world. I had yet to learn the importance of humility and heart posture—or even the fact that the Jesus I didn't know said stuff like this in the first place.

I figured the first step in becoming an adequate person would be learning socially acceptable communication—which had always been a peculiar concept, dispatched on an ongoing mission to elude my grasp. I could be fully determined to be talkative and give myself all the pep talks in the world, telling myself I was definitely going to stop being the quiet girl. The problem is that one of two things usually happened:

1.  I started losing control of my words the instant I began speaking, either in the form of completely butchering my eloquent, mentally rehearsed lines, or in blurting out something else entirely—often the first random thing that popped into my sorry head.

2.  Language all but abandoned me, turning the art of conversation into an advanced game of Whac-A-Mole. All I could do was awkwardly stand frozen, trying to keep up and becoming dizzier by the second, unable to slam the mallet down until long after the game ended.

Properly speaking with other humans was evidently something I wasn't capable of, given the unfailing brain glitches every time an opportunity presented itself. Those rare few who tried to be nice and reach out would always regret it because of the painful awkwardness that followed as I floundered, trying to act like a person on such short notice. I would occasionally force myself to do something that felt completely unnatural and attempt to initiate conversations with classmates, especially at the fresh start of a new school year, only to have them immediately turn to literally anyone else in range and talk to them instead. I exuded an awkward aura before I even said anything.

Or maybe I scared people with my stimming. Perhaps it was clearing my throat, twitching my eyebrows and blinking repetitively, obsessively popping my knuckles, whispering echolalia to myself (repeated words or phrases—a common autistic trait), or something I wasn't even aware of. Regardless of the reason, it seemed I was just a giant can of human repellent. I was okay with that up until a point.

Whether or not it was true, I honestly felt that it was only me. I would observe my peers rather intensely, and no one else ever seemed to struggle with social interactions like I did. There were popularity tiers, sure. But no one was friendless. No one had the kind of speech impediment that I had.

"You know what your problem is? You're too quiet and need to talk more!"

There's a pause as I try to carefully and thoughtfully craft a response to explain that it's not that simple without being rude.

*Let's see . . . Oh! I've got it!*

"That's stupid."

*Nailed it.*

You've now witnessed a day in the life of my childhood self. Whatever magical power I possessed to draw unwanted attention to my quietness, particularly from adults, my hushed presence always seemed to call out like some kind of homing signal to onlookers. It was as if I had the message, "Please give me the same, unsolicited advice every time you see me, permanently etching it into my brain and making a big show of it so I can never live it down," emblazoned on my forehead.

Just talk more. Say more words. Piece of cake—except for the part about finding words in the first place, as well as the mental strength to utter them. That's before all the countless unspoken rules and the fact that no one was interested in what I wanted to talk about. I've always held the common autistic trait of not liking small talk or having to be fake.

Kids at school could be talking about a pool party they were having that weekend. Determined to talk more, I'd approach them, take a deep breath, and start blabbering about a flash game I found on the internet. I accomplished my mission of saying words. I did not accomplish my mission of being liked.

If I was going to be given a hard time either way, I preferred to be in my comfortable default state of quiet while it took place.

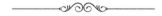

*I don't care what they say about me. I don't care what they think. Don't care, don't care, don't care. So why is it all I can think about? Why is it eating away at me?*

When I realized I couldn't really do much to renounce my awkward ways and be "normal," bitterness took over as the ruler of my heart. My internal rage continued to expand and spread as I got older, turning into a dwelling place that I'd call home. Unlocking the door, I dusted some cobwebs and unpacked my boxes, slowly acclimating to the darkness. Given enough time, even a murky cave can start to feel like a comfortable, cushioned fortress. I decided that if the world was going to ostracize me no matter what, I would hate people—passionately. Even if you didn't wrong me in any way, I would automatically assume you saw me as trash because that's how it always seemed to go. If you were nice to me, you had to be faking it. I didn't have to feel guilty about being mean because they were all going to hate me, regardless. I didn't have to try to be friendly, since it would undoubtedly be pointless in the end.

I knew this wasn't right but didn't care anymore. I chose to live for myself in a continual state of anger and self-pity.

*Hatred. This is easier. This protects me. I like it.*

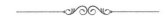

Here's some actual footage of my internal monologue at fourteen:

*I hate life. I hate people. I hate school. I hate myself. I wish I could just die. I hate everything. Life is pointless, since we're all gonna die, anyway.*

Whether it was the most minor of annoyances or something that really struck a sore spot, anything would set off that script. I'm told a lot of teens have those kinds of hyperbolic thoughts and that it's a phase. But I meant them. I lived by them.

I would meditate daily on how much I despised the world. It was especially intense during my first year of high school—my darkest days to date. I'd get so angry about my life that I'd contemplate punching through mirrors, despite my extremely low pain tolerance. Was it too much to ask to hide in my room for the rest of my life?

My personality was only one force to be reckoned with, as regular comments along the lines of, "You're ugly and fat, pumpkin face! When are you gonna do something about that?" made it clear that the ugly girl staring back at me in the mirror wasn't a perception limited to my own opinion.

Recall the image of the confused hippie from earlier and put her into the context of the fat-phobic culture that was much stronger a couple of decades ago. Evidently, all of my value was determined by my weight.

It was time to get down to business. Time to stop eating food unless it was explicitly non-fattening. So, fruits and vegetables only, forever, even though they nauseated me. It was crucial that I hit the gym every time I could successfully beg an adult to take me and jog in place obsessively when no one was looking. There wasn't a moment to waste.

Through vigorous efforts and highly questionable methods, by my early teen years, I had dropped a significant number of pounds within a few months—despite my stubborn, basically nonexistent metabolism that always refused to be a team player. As a bonus, I felt even more weight lift off my chest when I stepped onto the kitchen scale one day. I was finally in the 130s. I was elated and ready to face the world—that is, until an adult family member loudly commented, "You're 138 pounds? Wow. You're getting *fat*."

As a young kid, I was always told that I would grow up to be attractive. As a tween, I was told that I was a disappointment for not being attractive. This was hammered in extra firmly when another relative took my cousin and me to a fast-food joint of his choosing. He asked what we wanted as we walked in.

"I'll have a bacon cheeseburger," my cousin said.

"I'll have the same," I echoed.

"No! You're not allowed to have that, Miya!" our suddenly angry relative shouted.

"Why not?"

"Look at you! I'm *so* disappointed! You were supposed to be pretty!"

Shortly thereafter, I set off on my mission to become skinny, hoping that I could appease the world and fulfill my apparent destiny.

Sometimes, I legitimately tried to be healthy. Other times, I was living off two granola bars a day. It went on long enough that the school lunch lady recognized me and handed them to me before I said anything. But of course, I reported that I ate a big, proper lunch when asked. So don't feed me anything unless it's salad—and by salad, I mean plain lettuce. (Reader, please don't ever do this.)

But hey, I was becoming thin(ish); getting what I thought I needed. Did I become a different person and change my social ranking? In truth, I was mentally worse off that year than ever before. Changing your appearance, whether by safe and healthy means or not, doesn't magically give you a new brain. Upon returning to school the following year, the other kids didn't care in the slightest that I'd lost weight. As it turns out, it was never actually about that. A thin body is not, in fact, the equivalent of the mysterious social standards rule book that I never received. I know. I was surprised, too.

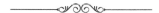

Childhood was filled with a constant back-and-forth desire between desperation to grow up and never wanting to. Freedom to do whatever I wanted sounded nice, but I wasn't ready for the "final boss" yet and doubted that I ever would be. Life was one of those games best left on the apparent easy mode that I could hardly handle as it was.

The consistent message I got from those older and wiser than me was, "If you think life is hard now, just wait until you get older." Life was always going to be a drag and would only get worse. I needed to work hard and be successful so that life could still be a drag. Cheers.

Thinking about the future in any capacity was terrifying. I didn't know how I'd ever last out there in the world—assuming I didn't get eaten alive first. Life was like traveling through a dark, forested labyrinth in the middle of the night with no map or like trying to navigate the Lost Woods from the *Legend of Zelda* games, though everyone else was far better equipped for the journey than I was. They had their huge backpacks full of supplies, compared to my nearly empty grocery bag, with its contents spilling out of the holes. Whenever I fell into a ditch and cried out for help, I went unheard because everyone else was too loud. I was a mere cricket in the middle of a sold-out rock concert; whether or not I made any noise didn't make a difference. I'd have to climb out myself, only to be yelled at and punished for being too slow and falling behind, probably because I was lazy.

I often wonder how differently things would have played out if there had been someone to tell me that this was all a normal part of being autistic and to offer appropriate support. I wonder how much richer those years would've been if someone had explained God and His unbiased, unconditional love in a way that I could understand. I'm thankful that neurodivergence is becoming much more well-known and being talked about. Hopefully, the world will feel less like the Lost Woods to future generations of autistics.

Back then, it wasn't nearly as socially acceptable to talk about mental illness and disabilities as it is now. It was generally viewed as enormously shameful. I don't doubt that had everyone known back then that I'm autistic, I would've spent my entire childhood being infantilized. I shudder to imagine what else. I wouldn't dare have opened up to anyone about my struggles that made me seem weak—especially with my mortifying speech impediment.

# CHAPTER FOUR
## The Great Internet Escape

I never thought this day would come, but it's here. Thunderous cheers erupt below as I step onto the stage in a sudden surge of confidence. The band is playing the opening instrumentals behind me. From every direction of the arena, all eyes are fixed on me as I grab the mic, ready to blow minds. Normally, it would be terrifying to be watched so intensely, but this is different. All the attention is positive, and I know exactly what I'm doing.

Who would've ever thought that loser Miya, of all people, could sing and had so much hidden potential? All it took was throat and jaw surgery to change my voice and fix my speech.

I recognize several faces in the crowd. People from school look up at me in awe—people who mocked me and all but walked straight through me on a daily basis. They were all just so impressed by the unexpected plot twist of my life that they now want to be friends.

The lights change colors as the drumbeats speed up and the crowd starts headbanging. I feel fire coursing through my veins as I fall to the ground in a moment of passionate belting, lost in a maelstrom of emotion.

Everything worked out in the end. People care about who I am. My life means something to the world. As I sing dramatically about pain, everyone who knows me is filled with empathy, and they all vow to never treat weird kids poorly again.

It's worth mentioning that this is all happening entirely in my head.

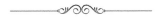

The year was 2007. As much as I would've loved to have been rocking out on stage in front of adoring fans, I was still living the proud shut-in life. That was okay because the game *Pokémon Mystery Dungeon* came out and became my biggest hyperfixation—perhaps the only source of joy that sparked life in me in spite of my circumstances. The game's primary themes of community and unfailing friendship made for a deep and tear-jerking plot—and a lot of hours.

One uneventful summer afternoon, I was playing this wonderful creation from the heavens and was stuck on the harder levels in the post-game. While I wasn't super familiar with the internet yet, outside of simple flash games, and largely associated search engines with homework, it occurred to me one day to make life easier and look up gaming tips.

Learning the true usefulness of Google for the first time, I ended up stumbling upon a website full of cheat threads and game discussions. The site basically doesn't function anymore, but it was an active chat forum back in the day. I went in expecting game discourse but found that people were just hanging out and talking about random stuff. That wasn't what I was looking for, but it intrigued me. It appeared that we shared some special interests, and I wanted to be part of the club. Hence, I created my very first internet login and invited myself into the chat.

The first thing I did in this exciting new community was attack people, starting a bunch of drama with a few individuals who seemed mean based on maybe two or three posts. Painfully cringe-worthy doesn't even begin to describe my behavior. I, the new girl who joined five minutes ago, was telling those people *they* should leave the community because I didn't like them. Then I aggressively made sure everyone knew that I loved cats—a lot. It was important information. But after all of that, I somehow befriended a bunch of those kids—the ones I didn't cause drama with, anyway.

To the victims I terrorized: if you happen to be reading this, I apologize from the bottom of my soul. Can we pretend that never happened?

Not to worry, I had the concept of internet stranger danger hammered into my head, so I was careful and didn't use my real name for the first year or so. Coming up with an alter ego was a whole mission. You should know that I constantly talked about how much I loved Miley Cyrus and her show, making it a well-known fact to an even greater extent than my love of cats. I knew my fake real-life name needed to be convincing, leaving absolutely no room for suspicion. So, naturally, I went with Miley.

I'm not sure if anyone actually bought it, but they all kindly went along with it. It was immediately obvious that we were all around the same age with the same interests, with everyone's extensive gaming and pop culture knowledge being perhaps the biggest indicator. I thought these people were the coolest. They regularly had me cackling with their unique senses of humor. How could real, non-TV humans possibly be so witty?

Admittedly, much of the "humor" was literally just saying random things, like "Sparkly dodos eating pizza and invading a coffee shop with a llama!" and sometimes having contests over who could be the most random. But as a tween, I thought it was hilarious, top-tier comedy. Of course, we always talked about real things, too, in a much less silly manner.

Little "Miley" ended up coming clean the following year. I told them my real first name and the kind of person I really was: an awkward, lonely loser with no life. This was after a year of trying to sound impressive by claiming that I had an amazing social life (and somehow also managed to reserve a thousand hours a day for internet chatting), even creating names and character profiles for my supposed real-life friends to sound extra convincing. So the reveal wasn't a casual or easy decision. I felt guilty for deceiving the only friends I had, so I made a big, dramatic confession. And to my overwhelming relief, they loved me all the more for it. I continued to fall deeper in, caring less and less about anything else.

At the end of the game that led me to the forum in the first place, the player chooses to stay in that world with their new community, never to return home. In an attitude of solidarity, I wanted to remain in this online world forever with my new friends, never to return to the real world.

We eventually upgraded and moved to an old-school social media website with an anime style. I loved the aesthetic and all the fun customization and games, especially since it meant I could flaunt my superiority and how "rich" I was through my extravagantly dressed avatar. Silly amateurs would undoubtedly cower before my might. It was all way more exciting than just a chat forum alone, even though that was the most important part.

I became desperately attached to that group of kids, taking immense comfort in being able to hide behind a computer screen and communicating solely by typing. They never had to know about my gross voice and speech impediment, and they would never know how awkward I was in person because these relationships were purely digital. I felt safe in that way. But despite being on a mission to keep my flaws a secret even after the initial confession, I got to a point of trust where I could share my honest struggles with some of them and not feel judged. They would support me instead of belittling my problems. Who knew that was a thing in life?

This was especially true of Melanie. Out of all of them, she was the one I loved the most and trusted more than anyone else in life. It's an invaluable gift to have someone in our lives who can lift our spirits in any and every circumstance, someone full of compassion and humor to whom we can relate deeply to and whose love for us stands strong even in the darkest of times—that's the person Melanie was to me. I was free to be myself every moment, fully confident that I was safe in doing so. It didn't matter that we hadn't met in real life or that we never had a conversation outside of a screen. She was my best friend in the world, and I proudly proclaimed that every chance I got. I may have looked like a loner in real life, but I had her. No one could see it since it was a long-distance friendship. But for the first time in ages, I wasn't friendless.

"You're not my friend! You're just my stupid sister!"

With that encouraging news in hand, I was dragged into a new chapter. It wasn't long after the divorce when one of my parents remarried. I turned thirteen, blinked my eyes, and became one of six kids in a loud, bustling household.

We were relatively, theoretically close with this soon-to-be-family beforehand and stayed at each other's houses frequently, so it didn't feel like the most dramatic change in the world. But it still took its toll. Even at a young age, I perceived a lot of fakeness and manipulation from the new family additions, with the exception of my new stepparent—which is ironic, since many autistic people tend to struggle with picking up on this kind of thing. But everyone told me I was being dramatic, so I just let it go for the time being. My stepparent was nice, so it should be fine. Probably.

"I feel like you don't care that I'm alive," was what I had told Shannon, my new stepsister with whom I would soon be sharing a room, at our parents' wedding reception. As usual, I couldn't find the words I was looking for but was being forcefully pushed by some relatives into having a talk with her against my will. What was supposed to be closer to, "I feel like you disregard my feelings and needs, don't respect my boundaries, constantly put me down, and shove me into a corner," just came out as, "I mean, you threw scissors at my face the other day."

This forced confrontation happened after I spent hours pouting, dying to leave. The room was bright and happy, with flowers everywhere and people laughing and dancing to upbeat music. And then there was the one angry child. One could visibly see the dark storm cloud floating above my head, complete with the occasional lightning bolts.

My comments to my new stepsister were brushed off, much like every other concern I had throughout this season. Everyone carried on with their business. I just needed to accept my fate—another reason to hate life. That entire wedding trip was a mix of overwhelm, internet withdrawals, and a deep sense of impending doom.

One night, while trying to fall asleep on the floor at some new relative's house, I started attacking my arm with random things I found under the bed in a fit of anger. I felt like a prisoner and a complete misfit in this new family, and there was nothing I could do about it. This was the first time I desperately wished that I could run away and move in with one of my online friends. We were only teens, but maybe one of them needed a roommate?

I spent that trip imagining scenarios where Melanie would somehow show up there and rescue me. The impossibility of it added fuel to my lonely, burning frustration. Whether or not it was true, I felt like the least important child in that household for years to come. If one of the six were to leave, I was confident in assuming they'd still be perfectly happy with five kids.

The new family members were brilliant actors. I was actually pretty envious. I could probably fulfill my then-dream of becoming famous if I had those acting skills, and I low-key wished they'd mentor me. Even when I saw through their façade toward everyone, it was still somehow convincing. But I did consider that perhaps I really was being too negative, that any poor treatment toward me was my fault.

Even though I recognized the fakeness and was skeptical, I still grew to trust them, as was my natural autistic tendency. I wanted to trust them, so I gave them all the benefit of the doubt, over and over. To be sure, we did have a lot of fun, memorable times together, whether it was at the dinner table or on the many family trips we took. The six of us would always ride our bikes to the grocery store and skate around the neighborhood. We spent many evenings battling each other on racing games. Movie nights were a frequent occurrence. They all had amazing senses of humor, easily able to make me laugh and lift my mood, even when I was in my dark state. They were some of the wittiest people I've ever known. For better or worse, I really looked up to them.

All the same, when I was around them, I felt incredibly small, especially around their extended family in big gatherings. There was no way I could compete with their energy and wit. Being the designated scapegoat, I got pretty clear impressions from some of them that they actively wanted me to know that I was an unwelcome misfit—as if I wasn't already aware.

My social struggles and overwhelm became public property for the whole family, always freely on display against my will, with an attached sign that I didn't approve that said, "Leave a Review." I wasn't allowed to object, as that would basically be a death sentence. Hence, my awkwardness and insecurities turned into a circus. It wasn't uncommon for us all to be hanging out and my biological parent randomly calling out at a volume that might as well have been through a megaphone, "Hey, Miya! Don't forget what we talked about the other day!"

"Oh? What did you guys talk about?" all the other kids would ask like eager puppies.

"We talked about how Miya needs to get a clue in life and stop being an embarrassment!"

There was also the classic dinnertime activity. "Hey, guys, because we care and we're all about positivity, let's play a game where we attack and eviscerate your sister! It's okay because we're joking. Come on, Miya, quit being so depressing! We're gonna keep doing this until you smile and laugh!"

One of the younger kids would come up behind me and bang on my head with their hands as hard as they could like a bongo drum. My head throbbed. My ears rang. Everyone laughed. I was supposed to laugh. But all I could do was muster every ounce of strength to suppress my rage and prevent an explosion that would obliterate the room.

"Come on, Miya! Smile! Cheer up! *Or else.*"

*I hate you all.*

I'd take a deep breath, retreat to my room the second I was allowed and claim to be doing homework when I was really talking to Melanie as she helped me calm down. Deep breaths. It was going to be okay. And then the doorbell would ring.

Those kids would regularly have friends over at our house, which was a completely valid thing. The problem was that, far more often than not, I would be forced to hang out with the girls, even though they wanted nothing to do with me and vice versa. Sometimes, I was quite literally pushed toward them after they walked through the door. Some of them were nice, but I imagined it probably felt like having their plans ruined so they could babysit some incompetent girl and make sure she was being social, per the orders from the adults. I didn't want to ruin their plans. But I wasn't given a choice, lest I risk getting in trouble and losing my computer privileges. I'd jump into a den of hungry lions before I'd ever let that happen. Shannon's change in demeanor the minute the adults walked away was all the confirmation I needed that I was unwanted. I just had to grin and bear it, with the reality looming over my head that I didn't fit in anywhere, even at home where it was supposed to be safe.

However, even in my black hole of a heart, I was still being protected by God—my Real Parent—unbeknownst to me at the time. I could've had violent meltdowns. I could've snapped at them all with my true feelings and been kicked out of the house. But I was never carrying my burdens alone.

If I could time travel and have a word with my past self, I would tell her that these people's opinions of her were trash because God would strongly disagree with them and He's always right. No person is any more or less valuable than another, regardless of external performances. He would know, considering He's God. I'd want her to know that she was never truly a loner to begin with. "'This is my command—be strong and courageous! Do not be afraid or discouraged. For the LORD your God is with you wherever you go'" (Josh. 1:9). She could've really benefitted from hearing that.

Instead, I naively believed that Melanie was my salvation in this life. As soon as I could get away, I'd run to her for support. She always had it readily available, making the precursory suffering worth it.

---

Preceding the internet days, there were brief times when I did temporarily have a couple of real-life friendships—if that's even the correct term. But they were either physically aggressive or into scary things that sent a certain terror through me. There was one who would frequently, quite literally, spit in my face for fun. As desperate as I was for friends, I felt like I needed to cut out these people—or, rather, freeze them out until they got the message, since I couldn't do confrontation. Once I got to a place of burning hatred toward humanity, I didn't even feel bad about it.

Melanie was different. I'm sure if she were a real-life friend, she never would've tried to wrestle or spit on me, and I would've appreciated it. But in all seriousness, I thought she was so mind-blowingly awesome and intelligent and hilarious—a true legend. The fact that someone as amazing as her would even give me the time of day was revolutionary, especially after my embarrassing confession about my life.

"Are you sure you don't hate me?" I asked her. "I lied to you and everyone. :("

"Not at all! *Hugs* I'm just happy you told the truth. I'm proud of you. :D"

Regardless of how weird I was being or how much I complained about everything under the sun, I knew she loved me no less and would always offer all the encouragement she could give. That would go both ways, though I hardly felt adequate to comfort and encourage by comparison. Other times, we'd just say random, silly stuff to each other and be total goofballs. A bad day could be easily turned around after talking to her. She called me her best friend as well, which was a title I took very seriously.

At the same time, it felt impossible. There was supposed to be nothing likable about me. The only people who said they loved me did it out of obligation because we're related but made it clear that they didn't like anything *about* me. But this top-tier girl actually enjoyed my company and was always willing and eager to come to my defense. Frankly, that in itself was a miracle that I'm surprised didn't lead me to God sooner.

"You had a bad day? *No!* I'll send you some funny pictures and virtual Skittles!" she'd say. Or, "Someone was rude to you on here, too? What's their username? I'll rate them down! >:)"

She always had my back, whether I was being given a hard time online or offline or needed to vent about my life and self-worth issues. Much of the time, I was just painfully lonely and needed someone to laugh with. I felt unworthy of her kindness but, nevertheless, took as much of it as I could get.

There were still some others from the group who hadn't left our online space yet, all of whom I loved as well without a doubt. But for some reason, I gravitated toward Melanie. Maybe it had to do with my autistic brain's hyperfixation tendencies, always zoning in on a limited number of things. I can't say for sure.

My inevitable addiction to my computer screen was growing stronger by the day. Logging on to talk to Melanie and the others was all I cared about— the only genuine positivity I had in my life. We didn't have smartphones back then, so I always had to wait to get on an actual computer. I hated waiting with every fiber of my being.

Family members always gave me this motivational speech: "Hey, lazy bum! Why are you *still* on the computer? You've got a problem! Lazy, lazy, lazy. Get off and go do something useful, or come spend time with the rest of us."

What I wanted to say was, "Why? So you can all judge me and say horrible things to me, playing them off as jokes and thinking I can't tell? So I can put on a forced happy act just so I don't get yelled at and punished? No thanks. I can't believe you're so dense that you honestly think I'd enjoy that. I want to spend time where I'm validated and genuinely wanted for who I am, weirdness and all."

What I was allowed to say was, "Okay."

Chatting with my internet friends was the only thing that mattered. Things I had previously enjoyed became sources of fury because they took me away from the one thing I cared about. Even going on vacations to fun places sent me into an internal tantrum, since it meant I would be separated from my beloved internet during that time. Though I wasn't allowed to say it, I would've been much happier if they had gone without me, leaving me at home in peace to go on online with no one to harass me about it.

We could be at some sort of fun local event, like Christmas lights or a New Year's festival, where everyone else was cheery. I, on the other hand, was a full-fledged grouch, going through withdrawals whenever I was away from the computer. I'd want to scream from the stress of potentially missing a good discussion thread because I was stuck at some obligatory outing.

This website wasn't just a special interest. It was an all-consuming addiction that I likely would've refused to go on living without. There was no joy in anything that wasn't the internet. I became that bitter, sulking grouch every moment of every day—not just when I was having a bad day to begin with.

It made sense, though. The digital world was like an alternate universe—one that didn't exist solely in my head. I didn't have to keep quiet. I didn't have to worry about pronunciation. I could take my time, think before I typed, and proofread my comments to filter out stuff I would've regretted less than a second after it left my mouth in a real-world dialogue. I could Google things if I didn't know what something meant or didn't understand a joke, and no one would ever know. There was nothing to worry about in terms of social and sensory overwhelm. This life was so much easier. I wasn't in as much danger of being judged or mocked. Excluding the trolls and a few individuals I instigated drama with, people would only say nice things to me. This is why the internet often feels like a much safer environment for autistics. When we're receiving less-than-stellar treatment from the real world but find online spaces where we thrive, it stands to reason that we'd gravitate toward the latter. I was just lucky that I didn't meet any dangerous individuals with sinister motives.

# CHAPTER FIVE
## The Best Friend I Never Met

**To:** Mel_9018

**From:** MiyaFire_827

*I hate my life!*

*Not only is IRL the worst, but even people here keep changing and I hate it! It's like I have to be perfect all the time otherwise they're done with me :(*


**To:** MiyaFire_827

**From:** Mel_9018

*I know!*

*I hate the way they changed :/*

*Why must they act so serious?*

*Being serious is BORING! D:*


**To:** Mel_9018

**From:** MiyaFire_827

*Right?! I'm just glad I have you. I know you'll never be like them. <3*

*I just wish I had at least one person IRL to hang out with and share everything with and all that. And you'd be the perfect one.*

*Sorry, I know it sounds corny.*


**To:** MiyaFire_827

**From:** Mel_9018

*Doesn't sound corny. I think it's sweet ^_^ I'd love that too.*

I was a freshman in high school at this point. Shortly before the semester started, Melanie lovingly encouraged me to join her in solidarity and adopt the "scene" style (which was basically emo but bright and colorful and a little less gothic). But only if I wanted to, of course. And I actually loved the idea. If she thought it was cool, that meant it was *cool,* no question. Anyone who disagreed was wrong.

It was an opportunity for a whole new image. Maybe with such a dramatic change, I'd be less invisible. Lots of the popular kids at school sported that style, after all. I didn't really understand it, but I'd have Melanie as a scene mentor to help me whenever I needed.

I had my long, unruly hair chopped off and dyed darker with a blonde streak, based on a random scene girl image I found. Naturally, my wardrobe didn't match the style yet, but it got there slowly. No more old man polo shirts combined with big, frilly skirts and flip-flops. Those days were over. I did my research on how to become a scene girl and tried my best not to come off as a poser. That's the last thing a scene kid wanted.

Scene rule number one: never admit to being a scene kid—except that was the one rule I was willing to break often. The world needed to know. My style consisted of uncomfortable skinny jeans, cutesy hair bows, graphic tees, choppy layers of hair, bead necklaces, coon tail hair clip-ins, checkered shoes, heavy makeup, and bracelets up to the elbow. I went all out. It was the law. Even though it took hours to tame my crazy hair, I still got up before sunrise every morning to do it. Scene kids had to have straight hair. I needed to mimic Melanie in my typical autistic manner because I still evidently didn't know how to be a person.

Of course, my change of style didn't do anything for my social difficulties. Like with the weight loss, people didn't care. I felt like an idiot for thinking that I'd show up to school the next day, and everyone would say, "Wow! I love your fashion modifications! I want to be friends with you now!" I don't know what I was realistically expecting, but I was at least hoping for something.

As time went on and my bitterness continued soaring to new heights, I got more intense with it. The style shifted, until nearly everything was black. Raccoon eyes became my thing, to match my freshly dyed black hair. I filled in my lids with black eyeliner like they were shapes in a coloring book, hiding them behind my black bangs to match my black attire. In short, I became the complete embodiment of an emo kid. The people around me did not appreciate my new look. But then I gazed into the mirror. For the first time in my life, I genuinely thought I looked beautiful.

Of course, when asked if I was emo, I would shut it down and say, "No! I'm *scene!* Get it right!"—just like the scene rulebook told me to do, minus the admission to being scene. Except I was definitely emo, full stop.

I didn't cut in the traditional sense because physical pain terrified me, given my low tolerance for it. But I occasionally took to my arms and wrists with dull objects when I was really upset. Thankfully, no permanent damage was done, but those were intense moments of despair. I would've done anything to feel better and for someone to have genuine compassion when they saw me—to offer comfort in a way that wasn't condescending or give me some sort of magic to make me like everyone else.

I got in trouble at home for all my heavy black makeup, but I wore it anyway because I thought I was ugly without it and being dark was an urgent necessity. I wanted everyone to know that I hated life and people with the passion of a thousand burning suns. Except for Melanie.

If there was anyone for whom I felt genuine (platonic, believe it or not) love, it was her. I dreamed that she and I would meet in person someday. Then I could victoriously, vindictively face the rest of the world and say, "See? I have a *friend*! I wasn't lying! I really don't need any of you."

But as it would transpire, even having online friends and being more confident in my appearance left me feeling empty. It wasn't changing my real-life circumstances that I was trying to run away from. I was still miserable and feeling worthless, even with Melanie and a few others being nice and encouraging me. Despite my gratitude for that, it was never enough.

I think it goes without saying that while I always tried to be kind to my online friends, I wasn't exactly a nice person after a while. I was rude to people, cruel to my younger biological siblings on a regular basis, and low-key wishing suffering upon people I didn't like—so, almost everyone. I even became something of an online bully toward those I didn't consider friends, being strongly against allowing them to join the club. While I couldn't communicate my inner hatred very well in person, I felt infinitely bolder online to say nasty things and get into fights, just as long as I could hide behind that blessed screen. At one point, I even created a website listing all the people I hated (mostly newer users), usually for no reason other than the fact that they were new and I had a prideful sense of superiority. But if I was being honest, it usually wasn't personal; I just felt threatened by them. I didn't want them to invade my club and steal my friends away. I'd have nothing left.

Of course, the friend group was never mine to begin with, and I had no say in whether my friends talked to and befriended the new people or not. Seeing some of them appearing to have more fun talking with the newbies than with me was nearly unbearable. I knew it was only a matter of time before I was phased out completely.

Naturally, the time came when my other close friends, minus Melanie, started to leave the site because they were over it and wanted to focus on their real-world lives. I should've been happy for them, encouraging them like a good friend. Instead, I was enraged and usually made sure they knew it. My so-called love for them turned into hate in a matter of seconds after reading their goodbye announcements because everything had to be a personal attack—clearly they were leaving *me* behind, since I was the center of the universe.

"Fine! Go! I guess I mean nothing to you. I hate you now, and I hope your real lives fail. I don't need you anymore, anyway! Melanie's still here and isn't going anywhere, and she's all I need."

In a twisted way, I found actual comfort in sadness and anger. It was my place to hide and keep my heart safe, a place I could call home—or so I thought. Addicted to deep negativity, I couldn't really imagine having any other mindset after so long. I was becoming the decisions I was making.

Seeing happy people often irked me. I assumed their lives were simply phenomenal, that they had lots of friends who loved them, and that they didn't struggle with anything, ever. There was no other conceivable way they could be happy like that. It wasn't fair. I hated them and their happy lives.

One of my biggest pet peeves that made me want to punch these cheerful people was when they asked, "How come you're so quiet?"

How is one supposed to answer that, anyway? (Seriously, I still haven't figured it out. I'm open to suggestions.) I assumed they were judging me with all of their might, trying to cover up their mockery and condescension with smiles and high-pitched voices. No one wanted to actually know me—only what was wrong with me. I despised them all and wished *they'd* be quiet for once. While I wanted to tear into them in a mixture of sass and rage, I'd simply mumble, "I dunno."

But of course, in addition to the happy and peppy ones, people also angered me when they were upset. Apparently, I was the only one who was ever allowed to complain about life. From my point of view, they had friends who adored them and families who didn't strangle them. They could speak clearly and had social lives. Their existences weren't the absolute joke that I perceived my own to be. Therefore, they had no right to ever be upset. People weren't allowed to be happy or unhappy. There was no winning with me.

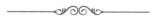

On a typical morning during my freshman year, I was sitting in the living room, waiting to leave for another dreaded school day. My hair was straightened, and my eyes were all raccooned up. Melanie would be proud. I was thinking about all the fun stuff we'd do if we met. Walk around the mall all day? Take selfies at the park? What do cool teens with social lives do for fun, anyway? She'd have to take the lead on that one.

A sudden lightbulb flashed above my head.

"Oh yeah, *God*. Huh. If He's out there, He's supposed to be all-powerful, right? Maybe I should pray that I can meet Melanie someday . . . and ask for a bunch of other stuff I want. Maybe if I give Him a big sob story, He'll feel bad for me and will grant my wishes. Might as well try, right?"

I never really took the idea of religion seriously and couldn't remember the last time we had been to church. I knew nothing about God, other than that He had supposedly created the world and decided where people go when they die. I imagined Him as some guy with mystical superpowers just chilling up in the sky somewhere. I didn't know that He isn't a wish-granting genie. I didn't know that He's deeply relational, knowing me better than I could ever know myself. I didn't know He was right there with me when I was crying in hiding places and wallowing in pain every day, suffering *with* me. I only ever turned to Melanie for comfort.

But as the year went on, something started to feel off, like we were subtly drifting apart. Conversations began feeling empty and lifeless. She didn't seem happy to talk to me anymore. Cue the utter terror within me. What would I do if I ever lost her? The idea was inconceivable. I broke down several times just thinking about it.

Hence, I devised a flawless plan: I would say random stuff to her incessantly until her enthusiasm returned—without actually expressing my concerns, of course. No need to be dramatic or anything. I never got anywhere in life by being quiet, so I figured I needed to talk more—and then some more. If we were drifting, it must be my fault for not talking enough.

I clung to her with all of my being, desperate like never before. She was the closest thing I knew to God's love at the time, so I made her an idol—the god of my life who would save me from my solitude. This isn't fair to do to someone. Though it can be easy to forget, we're just people. The coolest people in the world are still not Jesus. To place that pressure on someone else is setting them up to fail—or to drive them away. Sadly, I didn't yet understand the concept of idolatry and ended up falling down to the bottom of my own ditch.

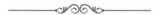

The day came when I couldn't take it anymore. I couldn't eat, couldn't sleep, couldn't think straight. I had been demoted from number one to number eight on Melanie's friends list, after all. Friend rankings on that website communicated a *lot*. I used that system as a way to flex my best friends while also conveniently being passive aggressive toward others. I was suddenly Melanie's number *eight*? What was that supposed to mean?

Leaving that knife in my gut for weeks led to me initiating something unthinkable: confrontation. I got up uncomfortably early that morning and sent my virtual best friend a message on a whim.

"Okay, Melanie. Tell me honestly: what do I mean to you?"

Waiting.

Waiting.

No response.

Still waiting.

The silence signaled the upcoming bomb on my life, and I refused to entertain the thought. I didn't have that luxury of denial for long, as a day or two later, I saw she had unfriended me. My heart sank into an abyss, though, at the same time, I wasn't all that shocked, which was shocking enough in itself. Perhaps it was the bloody dagger that was still puncturing it, but my gut was telling me that the worst-case scenario would happen. That day, my worst nightmare became reality.

*Everything is conditional. People will love you one moment and despise you the next. Nothing good ever lasts.*

# CHAPTER SIX
## Reason for Living Shattered

*Maybe it was a mistake. Maybe she was hacked. Maybe she was just making a new account like she always does and will add me on that one. There's no way any of this is real.*

I was sure that if I kept telling myself that, it would all work out in my favor. The site had an interesting system where if you unfriend someone, you still show up on their friend list until they also remove you. I sat there staring at the dreaded "they're on my list" message next to Melanie's username, telling myself over and over that it was a misunderstanding or a glitch. This whole thing would resolve itself.

I was fully aware that I was kidding myself, but there was nothing else I could do if I didn't want to completely fall apart and spend the rest of my life as fragmented pieces on the floor.

A couple of days later, my heart jumped at a notification. Melanie finally said something: "Take me off your friend list. And move on."

I did the healthy thing and pretended that hadn't happened, remaining in denial for a couple more days and making all kinds of excuses. I contacted a mutual friend of ours to see if she knew what was going on.

"No, she's been totally fine with me. She hasn't said anything about you."

Then Melanie came at me again with the familiar demand: "Take me off and get over it!"

This was the first time I'd ever felt actual anger toward her. I never thought I'd see the day. My face probably reached record temperatures as I impulsively replied with attitude, "Fine. Whatever. But first, tell me what your deal is. Why are you acting like this all of a sudden?"

"My deal? Fine, if you must know, I never liked you."

The sound of shattering glass could probably be heard within my chest. "You what? I get that you don't like me now, but *never*? Are you serious?"

"You were always clinging to me and driving me crazy," she continued. "I couldn't stand it. You're nothing but a nuisance. Don't get me wrong, I liked everyone else in the group, just not *you*. I'm finally moving on and making new, better friends. Now delete me and stay away from me."

I don't really remember how the rest of the conversation went, but those parts still exist outside of the blur. As strong as my denial was, the reality was there in those comments in plain, literal black and white, staring me in the face—until I deleted the comments because they were public and I was too embarrassed to leave them up for the world's viewing pleasure.

It wasn't just me being paranoid after all. Evidently, there's always a reason to be scared. This was my punishment for being vulnerable and trusting someone.

So that was it then. It was all a lie. Or she had come to a place of hating me so deeply that she made up this excuse at the end to ensure that she got rid of me. I'll never know.

*"You're so awesome! I love you, bestie!"*

Lies.

*"I wish I lived near you. Then we could be scene buddies! We'd have so much fun if we met! I'd make sure of it!"*

Lies.

*"People IRL don't like you? That's crazy. Who wouldn't like* you? *Well, in any case, I think you're great!"*

Lies, lies, lies.

I spent hours one night going through old comments and messages from back in the good old days when we were friends and she was always so kind and funny. It was a historical museum full of relics from the ancient past. Miya and Melanie: how the tragedy unfolded—for one of them, anyway.

I locked myself in my dark room and completely broke down. I sobbed my brains out but kept silent so my family wouldn't hear me. I wasn't about to allow them to have any part of this. If someone were to walk in, I would just pretend to be asleep. It didn't matter that I had finals the next day and would get my head bitten off if I failed them. The way I saw it, I had very little left to lose.

I was just a body—a waste of flesh that produces irritating noise called a voice, if not uncomfortable silence—a body that could've contained the mind and soul of the type of person my family and the rest of the world actually wanted, but it doesn't. I might as well conduct a lie detector test on everyone who claims to care about me—call them out on their deceit from the start and save us all a lot of time.

Life was a prison cell. Maybe every once in a while, I would get a fellow inmate to hang out with. They'd pretend to like me, and things would be a little better for a moment. But in the end, they'd leave, and I'd still be chained up in my dark, lonely cage—solitary confinement with my stupid, thick skull that never learns.

**MiyaFire827 posted a status:** *I can't do this anymore. It's over. I don't know what to do. I might just end it here.*

**To:** MiyaFire827
**From:** BlueNatalie5
*Miya, you shouldn't leave just because of Melanie. It would be awful if you decided to leave. I'm hoping from the friends who do love you that you stay and don't leave because of that one person.*

**To:** BlueNatalie5

**From:** MiyaFire827

*Well, I didn't mean just ending life online, if you know what I mean. Why does it have to be this way? What did I do wrong?*

Admittedly, there were still other friends like Natalie left who were wonderful, and I was very lucky to have them. But it wasn't enough for me. My source of hope and joy was taken away, and I couldn't see anything good anymore. With my heart's smoldering wick on its last leg, I figured I'd be left in my ditch to rot.

I'd also like to travel back in time to this moment and tell myself to look around. Look at the roof over your head in your safe neighborhood. Look at your full pantry and closet. Look at the gift of friendship you've found with several people in this online community that isn't limited to Melanie. Regardless of how things turned out, look at how much you learned from her and how you've grown through this season. Look at your sweet cats that love you. "Look at the birds. They don't plant or harvest or store food in barns, for your heavenly Father feeds them. *And aren't you far more valuable to him than they are?*" (Matt. 6:26, emphasis mine).

Amidst other people's crimes against me, I couldn't see all the ways God was providing and taking care of me, even down to letting me experience the desires of my heart through friendship. Losing my best friend was absolutely a valid reason for heartbreak and mourning. But even before that happened, I allowed myself to fall into a deep state of indifference toward all of the other rays of light in my life.

# CHAPTER SEVEN
## The Unexpected Invitation

Earlier that year, I had picked up longboarding before most people even knew what a longboard was. I wanted to be a skater like my then-favorite artist Avril Lavigne because that would absolutely make me cool and erase my problems, but I found that regular skateboards were too hard to navigate after a few gnarly wipeouts. It was much easier to not wipe out on bendy longboards, so that became my thing—even though I didn't, in fact, become cool or cause my problems to vanish with my newfound coolness. Massive bummer. Regardless, it was another fun distraction. Melanie thought it was awesome back when I had told her. That seal of approval was good enough for me.

Skating, music, internet, cats, a few nostalgic video games that I used to play with Matt—those were basically the only things I didn't hate or feel apathetic about in this season. But after losing the one thing I was living for, even that stuff couldn't do much for me.

It was the last day of freshman year. I had spent the previous night bawling my eyes out in the dark, but no one would ever know. I was supposedly switching schools the following year and not returning (which didn't end up happening, thankfully), and I hated the idea of change and uncertainty but didn't care enough to fight it.

My mind was an echo chamber. *If even my supposed best friend couldn't stand me after so long when she didn't even have to deal with me in person, what hope do I have? It's just going to keep happening over and over and over—that is, assuming I can even manage the overwhelming task of temporarily getting anyone to like me in the first place. I quit.*

I should note, I don't believe that I was actually suicidal. I had no plans or true intentions of doing anything—not yet, anyway. But if I didn't have my cats and maybe a couple of favorite songs and video games as special interests, perhaps I truly would have seen no reason to keep going. Perhaps down the line, I would have taken my life. I can't say for sure. At that point—and many times before that—I just wanted to disappear. I didn't want to see the light of tomorrow. I wanted to either be gone and have the suffering end (and make people feel guilty) or scream to the world at the top of my lungs and be noticed—really, truly noticed. I needed to do something that would allow me to be taken seriously.

Maybe that would look like dying. Maybe it would look like running away from home. Maybe it would look like magically becoming a famous emo rockstar with no voice or speech problems by some ridiculous miracle. The only thing I knew was that I needed someone to *see* me and empower me for who I was and not the ideal person they desired. Circumstances needed to change, but I had no control over that. I had already spent my whole life up to that point exhausting my own efforts.

Of course, the belief that absolutely no one on the planet liked me was a complete lie from the enemy of my soul. But I was too wrapped up in hatred, self-loathing, and ever-growing trust issues to see it any differently. I probably wouldn't have liked me either if I were someone else, so it seemed foolish to expect other people to. I was sure that I was unlovable beyond the surface and that no one would prove me wrong—no human, that is.

I didn't tell anyone offline what had happened with Melanie, especially at home. I didn't even need to because I knew how it would go. "Well, just get off the computer then! What have we been telling you all this time? Serves you right for wasting so much time, lazy bum! Live life in the real world like everyone else, idiot!"

And then I wouldn't be permitted to respond, "Don't you think I would've done that a long time ago if I could? That will never be possible for me. You should all know that by now. You can keep all of your condescending 'told you so' comments to yourselves. I hate you people. It's not like any of you have the slightest clue what it's like to be me. Must be *so* nice to be you."

I'd simply have to settle for a fake, "Sorry. Okay."

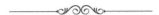

School was out for the summer. Everything was a blur. I did what I needed to do on that last day, whatever it was, then went home numb. It was going to be the loneliest summer break ever, if I even made it that far.

Oddly enough, instead of hiding in my room, I decided to go longboarding that afternoon. Maybe I could collect my thoughts and simmer down if I did something I didn't hate. Unlikely, but I figured it was worth a shot since I couldn't have my family getting suspicious and thinking something was wrong. An interrogation and lecture were the absolute last things I needed.

It was supposed to just be a casual stroll around the neighborhood on my board, like usual. I would only see a bunch of ugly brown and beige houses that all looked the same, with dehydrated, dying plants everywhere in front of gray brick walls. I would zone out, be sad, and suffer through the disgusting Arizona heat I hated so much. That's it. That was the plan.

I was not expecting God Himself to reach out to me there, changing my life forever. This experience, while dramatic in its own way, wasn't like a Paul in Damascus type of revelation. I didn't see the clouds part in the sky or hear God's voice roaring from the heavens like thunder. In fact, I didn't fully realize it was God right there in the moment, and it took my brain some time to catch up. But there's no doubt. It was subtle but had a certain weight to it.

I was out there skating in my usual pessimistic dwelling place: doom and gloom and woe is me. Life would always be brutal and pointless, and I was nothing without Melanie. Keeping my eyes on the road and all the ugly houses, shouldering more reasons to be sad than ever before, I mentally flogged myself for being so worthless.

Then there was a sudden shift. In the midst of my solo pity party, hope and positivity suddenly started coursing through me. A voice of reason gently took over.

"You've done everything you can in your efforts to save your friendship with Melanie. You've tried reasoning with her, you've tried talking with mutual friends, and you've tried waiting. But it's over. You can continue tackling this wall with full force, becoming more broken and beaten with each hit, but it's never going to break. Or you can get back up, walk away, leave that path behind, and start a new journey. A new life awaits you."

*Wait . . . What?*

"The choice to turn away from this path is there."

*But . . . I can't. I don't belong in the real world. And besides, I've screwed up so many things. I let things in my real life fall apart and die because I thought I didn't need any of it. How can I possibly fix it all?*

"You're not too far gone. This can all still turn around for the better. You *can* focus on life in the real world. It's your summer and your life. Melanie can't take that away if you don't let her."

I saw an image in my mind of a fork in the road, with a pretty sunset in the background. Though they both looked the same at the start, one path would eventually lead to destruction, and the other would lead to life. I was off to the side, crashed on a bike and injured. I had the option of staying there and rotting in that spot forever if I wanted. I could choose to continue down the destructive path. Or I could pull myself up, repent, and move forward on the path of life.

Then came the sudden, strong convictions of, "I need to have a relationship with God. I need to seek Him genuinely—not just when I want my wishes granted but for a real relationship with Him and to learn more about Him. I need to focus on that. It's the most important thing I could ever do."

*That's . . . that's true, isn't it?*

In that moment, I felt like a fool—not in a shameful way but in realizing what should have been obvious from the start. What was I doing all that time when I could've been resting in the Lord of the universe, Who was there all along? This was the opportunity of a lifetime.

*Okay. I'm gonna do it. I'm gonna pursue God.*

Nothing felt weird about the suddenness. Every fear of the unknown left me. These convictions left an essence that I can only describe as peace; a sense of knowing that this is *right*.

As I was cruising around on a four-wheeled piece of wood on that hot day, I made my decision. Melanie and the rest of the world would not rob me of my life. I was going to dedicate my life to the One Who gave it to me in the first place. It was there that my heart began to transform and a new season began.

Like I said before, initially I didn't recognize it as an invitation from God. For a moment, I kind of thought, *Wow, I just became a happy optimist and a people person out of nowhere. What a pep talk I gave myself! I suddenly want to live life outside of the internet and am not afraid. Good for me!*

The reality is that I had no intention, nor the ability, of changing on my own. Hatred and sadness were all I knew by then. A lot of first-person thoughts were thrown into the mix in that moment, as opposed to the kind of thing a lot of us expect with these experiences. It wasn't, "Hey, Miya, this is God, so listen up." But it was all convictions I never would've had on my own and a call to do things that went against my very nature, like loving and forgiving people who hurt me.

It was as if I truly came alive for the first time. I could see beauty in things that I hadn't before. There would be times when I'd look at something as simple as a tree and would be overtaken with joy. God made every minute detail of that tree. And He also made me.

Some things naturally took more time, but a lot of it was basically overnight. I didn't hate life or people anymore, though the latter took a bit longer in some cases. In fact, I almost immediately started honestly proclaiming in my heart every single day, "I love life! Life is good!"

No, really, I'm not kidding. And it was completely genuine. I would've expected this shift to feel like exercising, with the muscles of my heart screaming in protest through vigorous mental training to not be hateful and melancholy anymore. But there wasn't a trace of that.

I was able to move on from Melanie faster than I would've ever expected. One of the most obvious inexplicable things was how I suddenly became socially competent—to a degree. Awkwardness runs through my blood and veins, so of course, it was still there—but significantly less so.

I got along much better with my family for a while, despite everything. I became close with Shannon for a long time through an unspoken pact. I was genuinely smiling often. Even when things were less than ideal or I was in a difficult situation, I was filled with a joy that certainly doesn't come from this world. I was frequently looking up and smiling at God, giving Him thanks.

My siblings would sometimes notice and ask, "What are you smiling about? That's weird and kinda creepy." For once, I truly didn't care if I was weird. Let them raise their brows at me. I was so happy to be loved and ransomed by God.

When sophomore year started, I was ready. It was the first time in my life that I was stoked for school instead of wishing the planet would explode before the first day. I actually liked how black hair looked on me, but I didn't want to come across as dark and emo anymore. I proceeded to dye the back half of my head blonde to balance it out. (This earned me the nickname "Skunk Head" by certain family members. But, hey, I liked it at the time, and that's what mattered.)

In due time, I stepped back onto the campus that I thought I wouldn't see again. I'd previously had a few casual lunch buddies (though I'd used the term loosely). While I was thankful that I didn't have to reenact *Mean Girls* and eat in a bathroom stall, I had fully convinced myself back then that they didn't actually want me there. I thought they merely tolerated my presence because they didn't want to be rude. How wrong I was.

I acknowledged the possibility that they might not want to continue hanging around me, since I was a negative, standoffish, full-fledged weirdo. I was still going to take the leap, regardless. If all my efforts failed, I would trust God to help me make new friends, despite how scary it felt.

The warm, bright morning on the first day of school fit the mood. I saw the whole gang in the courtyard and went up to them with a smile and friendly demeanor.

Deep breath and . . . "Hey, guys!"

"Miya!" they called out. "It's so good to see you!"

They smiled at the sight of me. They greeted me with hugs. They accepted me as if nothing was ever wrong in the first place. They were stoked that I had the same lunch period. The amount of relief and gratitude that flowed through me was indescribable.

We became good friends, for real this time. Conversing with them felt much more natural and less strained than ever. I even began hanging out with them outside of school, which was unheard of. At school, we were all in the same space and people had no choice but to share the same air as me. For anyone to want to spend intentional time with me elsewhere was a monumental deal.

There even came a time where I was a little more open with some of them during awkward moments of silence, saying things like, "Sorry, I'm not the best at starting conversations. Sometimes, I just need a little help."

Thanks be to God, I was not put to shame or unfriended for doing so. I didn't think that kind of acceptance was possible outside of the internet. These amazing people were actually seeing my struggles and quirks in the flesh, and they still enjoyed my company. It wasn't fake or manipulative. It blew my mind.

I'd frequently walk out of class with a big, dopey smile on my face as I made my way through the crowds that no longer overwhelmed me. People probably thought I was thinking about some boy I liked. No, my head was about to burst with thoughts of, *I have friends! They're real! Thank You, Lord! I love them so much to this day.*

Being social and learning how to navigate conversations became more and more natural over time, until it was almost effortless. I was even making eye contact without being told to, and people noticed. I wasn't clingy and didn't feel the need to be. I finally felt like I was "normal," whatever that was supposed to mean. People who didn't know me back in the day wouldn't have ever guessed that I used to be a quiet loner who hated everything. This wasn't some act of superhuman willpower. God gave me a new heart.

I literally believed it to be impossible in the past. But as the years went on, I was hanging out with friends every day, pretty much every chance I got, being a temporary *extrovert* by some miracle and loving every moment of it. My past self would've wondered, *Who is that person? She looks like me, but that's undoubtedly somebody else. An impostor is on the loose, but . . . I like her better. She can stay.*

Hating people used to come so naturally. It was such an easy thing to do. But after I gave my heart to God, over time, I grew to love people so deeply. I loved them to the point of crying sometimes. I loved them even when they weren't so nice to me. I learned how to forgive and have grace for people's shortcomings and genuinely wanted good things for everyone. I actually cared about the lives of others and not just my own, and I wanted to be there for them during the bad times in whatever ways I knew how. Being hateful began to make me feel disgusting inside in a way I hadn't really felt before.

This was all God. He healed my bitter, tattered heart and took me on adventures I would've never imagined possible. I had been committed to staying resentful and miserable forever, but He made welcome changes to my schedule and turned me into a new person. I wouldn't be here a decade and a half later, being the person I am or writing about God and what He's done for me if it weren't a reality.

This all might sound like an unfair unicorn story to some. And I get it. But rest assured, it's not that simple. This season when things were suddenly easier didn't last forever; but we'll get to that later. In my very limited knowledge and extreme ignorance, I believed that all of this meant that my autism was gone. I believed that God "healed" me from it, due to all these dramatic changes. It would be many years before I learned otherwise.

Looking back, I'm grateful for what happened. I may have never come to know God if I hadn't lost Melanie. A lot of times, we wonder things like, "If God really loves us, why did He let *this thing* happen? Why does He allow for so much pain?"

To be frank, I'm not quite sure where I stand on the philosophy of "everything happens for a reason," and it can be an incredibly insensitive thing to say to someone either way. But I do think that in some cases, such as my own, things seem hopeless because we can't see the bigger picture. I could've spent the rest of my life wallowing in pain and bitterness, wondering why God allowed me to lose my best friend and let me suffer so much up to that point. But if that incident had never happened and Melanie and I had stayed friends, I wouldn't be who I am. For all I know, I could've ended up far worse off, even with her friendship, because she's not Jesus. It was never her responsibility to save me. I could have gone down a really dark path and never gotten off, wondering why even my favorite aspects of life weren't fulfilling me.

So even though I think it could've been done more nicely, I'm thankful for the loss and the suffering—and I don't say that lightly. I'm so much better for it. And ultimately, I think I needed more of a tough-love situation in order to really surrender and turn to God as my true Hope. If Melanie had friend-dumped me in a nicer manner, knowing the way I was, I likely would have still clung to the hope of us being friends again someday or would believe that she wasn't really serious or would change her mind. I wouldn't have let it go. I needed that firm, "No, I mean it. We're done." So while I don't ever think it's cool to talk to people the way she talked to me, I'm thankful. It was for the best.

I believe God allowed me to lose my idol and hit rock bottom so that my heart would be available and I would turn to Him instead. Why would I have done so otherwise in my stubbornness when my devout faith still belonged to someone else? He let me get to a place of humility so I would understand that I need Him and would get over my pride and be willing to follow Him, knowing that everything else in this world is temporary and will leave me empty and unfulfilled. Nothing and no one can take His place.

In terms of storytelling, it would be easy to end it here. Whenever I've told this story at church, this has always been my stopping point because it's a happy ending before things got a lot more complicated. But I believe those complicated, not-so-happy parts of our stories are crucial and don't get shared enough. What actually happens after "happily ever after," anyway?

In one of my favorite books, *Blessed Are the Misfits,* Brant Hansen discusses how we tell a lot of half-stories in church settings: "We get the 'victory' stories over sin and depravity, but no one publishes books called *Whoops, I'm Totally Messed Up Again.* That's where the stories of our actual lives are. But we don't like our stories open-ended. So we clean up our stories and act like they're finished. And we clean up ourselves and act like we're finished."[2]

Telling happy stories and *only* happy stories leaves a lot of people feeling alone or like they're doing something wrong. I would go on to feel that way in the years to come. So I want to share the messy stuff as well. I believe God's glory still shines in the hard times.

But first, there were some adventures.

# PART TWO
*Keeping the Faith*

# CHAPTER EIGHT
## Slowly Learning

It was late afternoon, and all was chill. My parent was watching some sitcom in the other room. Five-year-old Miya was derping around after her cousins had left from a playdate. Those cousins would often bring over toy cars, toy bugs, toy everything and this time was no exception. I noticed a colorful spider the size of my hand over by the stairs after they left. It had bright, almost neon orange and green stripes on its back.

"Oh, looks like the boys forgot one of their toys," I said to myself.

I went over to pick it up, and it jumped. At me.

*Nope, nope, nope, nope*—I screamed bloody murder as I sprinted over to my parent in the other room at the speed of light. I probably could've given Sonic the Hedgehog a run for his money.

"Help! Big, scary spider! It's gonna kill me!"

I don't know what my parent did and didn't particularly care. All that mattered was that the gargantuan arachnid did not live to tell the tale. I was safe.

I think about this incident sometimes, as I would much later come to realize that this is the attitude we should have toward God. It's a cheesy analogy, I know. But it's true. When we're scared, we ought to run to Him as a trusted Father, much like how many of us would run to trusted parents or other guardians for safety when we were very young and afraid—not because the church says we're supposed to but out of natural instinct.

Our family's church attendance had decreased in frequency over time until it was basically never, except for the two big holidays. We were CEOs (Christmas-Easter-Only), as my sibling always called us.

In seventh grade, I was forced to go to confirmation classes for a while. That was the thing for preteens to do, depending on what denomination you belonged to. I didn't get much out of that, either. I was still the space case who didn't talk and was having a lot more fun thinking about flying around on a dragon and destroying noobs in battle.

"So what did you learn in confirmation today?" one of my parents would ask me afterward.

"Uh . . . "

"You *were* paying attention, weren't you? You'd better have been."

"Um . . . something about Jesus being both God and a man? I think?"

"What else?"

"Um . . . "

I hated that I was being forced into extra school on the weekends and didn't understand why they wished to torture me so. Others clearly didn't value my precious free time like I did.

*So God is supposed to be this Supreme Being or something, and I feel like it would be some kind of ultimate disrespect if I said I hate being here. But . . . I hate being here.*

Little did I know that God loves honesty. It's not like He doesn't already know what's in our hearts.

By the time I made my own decision to be a Christian, the family had stopped going to church, other than on those big holidays or if my pastoral grandfather was in town. Though it was a bummer, I didn't want to ask that we start going again, knowing that all my siblings would probably hate me for taking away their Sunday mornings.

At first, I really didn't know what I was doing. What does being a committed Christian even look like, anyway? But a thought eventually occurred to me: *Oh yeah,* the Bible. *That's a thing. I should probably read it to learn more about God, right?*

I remembered the little Gideon Bible buried in my nightstand drawer that I was randomly handed outside my school one day and kept for some reason.

I started reading a chapter per night, starting with Matthew and . . . a list of names I couldn't pronounce. In all honesty, I really didn't understand most of what I was reading and didn't find it very interesting. The level of intrigue evoked was similar to that of reading a dense school textbook. But I kept at it anyway because I wanted to learn what I could, even if it wasn't much. It seemed like something that was pleasing to God. I knew it was worth it. I'd usually do it in secret, hiding in my room with the door closed, because I had a strong feeling I'd be given a hard time about it and just didn't want to deal with that yet. The whole "unashamed of my faith" thing wasn't yet a concept I was familiar with.

Over time, I was finding some wonderfully comforting nuggets in that little Gideon Bible that did make sense. I like to think that God was lovingly revealing Himself to me in small doses at a time at a rate I could handle.

"'Don't let your hearts be troubled. Trust in God, and trust also in me. There is more than enough room in my Father's home. If this were not so, would I have told you that I am going to prepare a place for you? When everything is ready, I will come and get you, so that you will always be with me where I am'" (John 14:1-3).

My junior year of high school was when I finally got plugged into a faith community. God brought a wonderful friend into my life the previous year, who I later came to find out was the president of the school's Christian club. It was the first club I was ever actively involved in, and I was thrilled to learn that a group like that even existed. I didn't know it was possible for other teenagers to be interested in church things and not just our parents and grandparents. I was stoked to connect with other people who loved Jesus and also to ask my millions of questions.

That began the process of really learning about God and the Christian faith. I realized more and more how little I knew, as even hearing the word "sin" on the first day shook my heart. It wasn't a word I'd heard often, if ever, before that. "Christ died on the cross for our sins." That's supposed to be the most basic and fundamental thing in Christianity, but I somehow had never really comprehended it or heard it put that way until then.

"God's love is *unconditional*," they would say. "That means it never changes, no matter what."

*Wait, seriously? Even when I mess up? Even when I'm the worst, His love for me never changes? At all? Not even a little? He won't ever walk away from me or give up on me?* I knew God was loving, but this still threw me for a loop.

I felt such a heavy weight lifted off my heart, knowing that I never had to worry about God changing His mind about loving me like people do. It's not about anything I could ever do or not do. Past, present, and future, He stays the same. I'd never annoy Him with my existence. I'd never have to worry about Him not understanding me. I'd never lose Him if I didn't meet a bunch of criteria outside of accepting Christ. I was secure.

On top of the fundamentals, just learning about the Bible as I was going through it myself and having others to help me understand it better over time was eye-opening. It was where I learned that the Bible is essential and not just some side thing. I've always struggled with interpreting tones over text, especially when there's a lack of emoticons, so hearing other people's perspectives was so valuable.

In addition to the Scripture deep dives, I learned that I'm still allowed to ask for prayer, even when I wasn't in as bad of a situation as the person sitting next to me. I learned that it really is important to live for God all the time, beyond just going to church on Sundays. I had a feeling, so it was good to know I wasn't imagining things.

It wasn't until my senior year that I started going to an actual church and got involved. I then learned that teen youth groups are a thing—ever so slowly catching up to speed with how church stuff works. I had always viewed church solely as a place to worship and not a social club. Upon meeting the youth pastor and later joining the Wednesday night Bible study, I became part of the social club. It turned out it was actually valuable to have fellowship.

Though it was similar to my school group, just the concept of a Bible study alone, and hearing it be called a Bible study, blew my mind. I could actually *study* the Bible with more people who share my beliefs and came to the group willingly. We were studying, even though it wasn't for school and we technically didn't have to. I didn't have to do everything by myself.

Lovely friendships were made in that group. I ended up impulsively getting involved in volunteer activities on Sundays. I spontaneously invited our youth pastor to speak at my school group a couple of times. It was like a crossover universe.

We went on a summer beach camp trip, along with some other churches, where I befriended a girl who was in my original confirmation class during my dark days. She told me multiple times that I was "so different" from back then and basically a new person entirely, to which I wanted to do a happy dance and say, "Yes! It's true! Look at what God did!"

When it was time to graduate from high school, the church hosted a "Senior Sunday" event to celebrate the new graduates. It was just me and one other person in the group graduating. It sounded like it would be laidback.

Then my youth pastor contacted me. "Hey, Miya. How would you feel about sharing a bit with the congregation for Senior Sunday this week?"

Good thing my fear of public speaking was still on its long vacation. Sure, I could give a quick, generic speech about school. No biggie. Then my eyes widened to the size of dinner plates upon realizing he wanted me to share my faith story. I'd never done that before. Would it be okay? Would anyone even care?

I started thinking of Lacey Sturm, the original singer of the band Flyleaf, of whom I became a massive aficionado starting that year. She's still my favorite. I even met her once for an entire thirty seconds after a concert, where I eloquently managed, "Uh . . . hi. Thanks for, uh, doing what you do . . ."

I had watched every video the internet had to offer of her testimony, and it blew me away every single time. Listening to her in light of this opportunity assured me it's okay to talk about my dark and ugly past and that it's not something to be afraid of. It would show that I'm a real human. Vulnerability will glorify God and help people connect with the story.

I went on to share my own testimony in the large sanctuary when that day came, though the short timeslot forced me to keep it brief. I hated how I could hear my ridiculous voice through the microphone but tried to ignore it. I figured people would zone out—or, at the very least, be annoyed by how I sound, likely struggling to make out everything I was saying due to the cursed speech impediment. But the number of people who came up to me afterward and said my story was inspiring sent a message I didn't know I needed.

Feedback ranged from, "Out of all the testimonies I've ever heard, I've never heard one as touching as yours," to, "I also suffered through depression in high school. Thank you so much for sharing," and "You had me tearing up! I love how conversational you were, not even using a script! Just speaking from the heart." My universe was shaken. These were people I'd never met before, coming up to me, shedding tears for me, and praying for me, even though we were strangers. They didn't know me until listening to me babble for a few minutes, yet they cared about my life.

I really thought about the concept of sharing testimonies after that. I'd do it again and again if I could. I decided that I wanted to proudly share my story whenever I got the chance with anyone who desired to listen because it *is* powerful. The workings of the Lord always are.

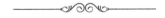

It was time for another family split. When other people started catching on to the stepfamily's fakeness and other concerns I initially had, things escalated quickly. My relationship with Shannon was the first to crumble. Even the nice stepparent turned on me the moment I made a weak attempt at something resembling standing up for myself.

There seemed to be a lot more to the parents' fights and reasoning for ending it, but I was still a child at the end of the day and wasn't given all the details. According to some, the whole thing was my fault, even though I was told by other adults to boycott the stepfamily and stop speaking to them. And so I did, in my own awkward way, because amid all the tension, my old frustrations were brought back to the surface. Despite our bonds, I couldn't go on ignoring the toxic chaos now that others were seeing everything. It all became real again.

I was sat down by various people and told some of the nasty things the stepfamily would say about me behind my back, with no punches pulled, and how constant it was. I was nothing but a mindless robot with no friends and a pathetic excuse for a human being. I could vanish into thin air, and they wouldn't care. It would make life easier and less embarrassing for them. Basically, they never really liked me.

That sounded awfully familiar. B.C. (Before Christ) Miya would have fallen into despair. B.C. Miya would have hated them and held grudges forever. B.C. Miya would have likely never trusted anyone ever again. This could've very well been what pushed B.C. Miya over the edge, possibly literally.

Instead, I clung to my Lord. It was a frustrating and devastating situation, but I never fell into a black hole. I didn't become a vicious, bitter person as I likely would have otherwise. I prayed. I placed my trust in God and found joy in Him. I held tightly to gratitude for all He's done for me. He was far bigger than the circumstance.

Ultimately, the split seemed to be for the best, due to all the toxicity, though maybe I'd feel differently if I went back in time and understood it all better. Maybe it wasn't all as bad as I made it out to be, or maybe it was even worse. It's easy to look back and wish I had talked through things more and been more of a peacemaker, but I was conditioned to just be submissive to orders from adults—but only the correct adults. Despite catching onto it early, I was still generally easy to manipulate by people I trusted. I wasn't all that great at discernment (and let's be honest, I'm still not, but I've gotten better. I think). If the "Good Guys," who were always the ones to be trusted, said that someone was bad and beyond hope, then that's what I got on board with. I was the first witness to a lot of the bad stuff in this case, so there was a prideful sense of vindication—something I had to surrender to Christ.

Regardless, I still pray for them and for any lingering bitterness in my heart to be destroyed. In the end, I never genuinely hated them or had ill will toward them. If it weren't for God, I would have no intention of ever forgiving anyone if they did me wrong.

# CHAPTER NINE
## Fear's Playground

Anxiety has been a part of me for as long as I can remember. I don't know if it's due to my upbringing, a comorbidity with autism, a random standalone thing, or perhaps a three-for-one combo. It's all I've ever known. This world has always been scary, and it boggles my mind knowing there are people in the world who *don't* worry on a near-constant basis. There are countless "what ifs" in life, after all.

For instance, what if I (or someone I love) get into a car accident? Develop some life-threatening disease? Become a victim of burglary? Lose everything and end up on the streets someday? Get attacked while out in public? Get bitten by a venomous insect while sleeping? What if I'm sealing my fate into stress-induced chronic illness at this very moment by worrying about this stuff? What if—

This is the operating room of my brain that I really wish would chill out and minimize production. I frequently go through a mental list of all the things I could fret about. I'd rather not say how long I believed that doing so was normal and healthy. Anything could happen at any time. I've gotta be ready! By being scared senseless. Over the years, I've been trying to work through all of this and put my trust in God. However, anyone who struggles with anxiety can attest that it's much easier said than done.

One of the first things the teacher said in my driver's education class was, "The whole point of this class is to scare you all so that you don't mess up on the road."

With that out of the way, we went on to be educated with gruesome stories of car accidents and graphic images and videos. They made it clear that no matter how smart and safe you are as a driver, your life is constantly in danger, and you could die at any second because you never know what idiotic things *other* drivers will do. Are you sure you need to make that trip to the store? Don't you know that every time you get into a vehicle, it could be your last moments on earth? Might as well kiss your life goodbye as you shut the door.

I mean, technically, that information wasn't incorrect, but it wasn't exactly fun to digest, especially since my family and I had to commute daily through a highway that was infamous for constant accidents. I wondered how anyone could possibly drive so casually without panicking every moment. Was I even allowed to sneeze or blink my eyes while driving without risking a crash? I procrastinated getting my driver's permit because I didn't trust myself with such a scary responsibility. And then there was the executive dysfunction when it came to studying for the test. But it was mostly the fear.

I didn't realize back then that not everyone struggles with anxiety like I do. I also didn't know that God tells us in His Word not to be afraid—and rightly so. Fear and stress over anything, no matter how rational it might feel in the moment, do nothing but spread like an electric poison through me until I'm a petrified pile of mush on the ground.

What happens on the road is one of those things that's out of my control, like many other things in life. Not many of us enjoy that feeling. I would go on to learn more and more with time that I need to trust God in all things, both out of obedience and for my own well-being.

But as mental illnesses like anxiety typically go, sometimes I can't do anything about it. Even knowing full well how irrational an episode of panic is while it's happening, logic doesn't matter in the moment. There's no magic switch for an extremely complex matter such as this.

I won't lie. Hearing people tell me to "just trust God" can be incredibly frustrating sometimes because it feels like the spiritual equivalent of telling someone who's having a panic attack, "Just stop worrying! Just stop thinking about it!" (Please don't ever say that, by the way.) It's as if they believe hearing someone say that suddenly makes anxiety go away or that I'd never thought of trying that myself. Yes, I've tried praying about it. Yes, I've tried going for a walk. I've done everything I'm supposed to do, but sometimes, it only wants to fight back. Sometimes, I simply need support from those around me as I ride the wave.

However, God is not like people who patronize us with clichés just to brush off the issue so that we'll shut up about it. He wants us to talk to Him about it. He can be trusted. It can be painfully difficult at times, in all honesty. I wouldn't dare deny that I struggle. I'm still working on it.

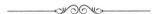

I was never one to believe in ghost stories as a kid, until I started hearing people I knew talk about their personal experiences. I couldn't argue with things they actually witnessed. All of a sudden, I felt like I was in constant danger of the supernatural. That fear wore off with time as I found distractions, only to come running back for a full assault years later.

Junior year of high school was right around the corner. One of my step-siblings had agreed to watch a popular horror movie along with my brother and me one night, promising to make goofy commentary throughout to lighten the mood. This step-sibling stayed for about one minute and then got distracted and left, but it was too late to quit. I didn't want to chicken out. That would be so uncool.

My response at the end was, "That wasn't so bad! Kinda boring, actually. Hardly anything was even happening for most of it."

But that didn't matter in my case because pretty much anything scary, regardless of extremity, is a major trigger—even if the effects are delayed. I knew this was an area of weakness for me, but trying to prove my supposed bravery felt more important. Being uncool ended up still happening, but like eight thousand times worse than it would've been had I just stopped watching in the first place.

A few days passed. It was getting late, and all was quiet. I was sitting in a dark room on my laptop, going about my usual business. Looking up, I suddenly saw a light flashing on the wall for a couple seconds and immediately got triggered. I couldn't just ignore it. That would've been too easy. Later on, I thought I noticed objects had moved while I was gone. I woke up one morning to the bathroom sink turned on when no one had been in there. I was suddenly hearing creepy static coming from my radio in the middle of the night. The first few things could've been someone trolling me, but that last one was a straight-up horror movie trope. The overthinking, catastrophizing anxiety monster within me joined the chat, quickly taking over the entire site like a hacker. There was no more room for peace or logic.

I believe that if there's ever something the enemy of our souls can use to torment us, he'll sadistically pounce on the opportunity. I probably would've normally ignored those weird things and forgotten about them. This time, my mind went straight to the movie, as well as every other scary thing I'd ever watched or heard about—all while swearing that my fears had nothing to do with the movie. It was happening at both my parents' houses, which meant it wasn't just tied to a specific place. It meant that I could be like the girl in the movie, having a demon following me everywhere because I was the target. I obsessed over it to the point of literally making myself ill.

As a newbie Christian, I didn't know anything about this stuff outside of what I saw in the small handful of movies I'd foolishly watched against my better judgment, as well as a few mentions in my slow progress through the Bible that I didn't really understand. But if it's in the Bible, it has to be true, right? I couldn't argue with that. So what was I supposed to do to get rid of this thing? Not even the priest could do anything in that movie!

Watching this kind of stuff in the past would have me thinking, *Surely if something scary were to ever happen in our house or if I told trusted adults that I saw signs of something supernatural, they would believe me and do everything they could to keep us all safe, right?*

You can probably guess where this is going. A large part of me always yearned for protection in general. I've always wanted to feel safe in every sense of the word. So realizing that I wouldn't be getting that from my family in this situation was like pumping steroids to my already-rampaging anxiety behemoth. I always wanted at least one other person in the room with me at all times, so there would be a witness if anything weird went down. Then maybe I'd be taken seriously.

For all of our safety, so we could all be on alert and figure out our combat strategy to take down the evil ghosts, I sat down with family members to discuss the whole ordeal. At first, they were surprisingly patient and listened to my concerns. Then they switched gears.

"Enough, Miya! There's nothing there! There's no such thing as Hell, no such thing as the devil, no such thing as demons. In this house, we don't believe in that stuff. It's all in your head! So be a good Christian like the rest of us and simply believe that God exists and just leave it at that."

"But the Bible says—"

"You don't need to read the Bible. Just believe in God."

I got a lot of mixed theology growing up, so that was a fun thing to wrestle with later on. I trusted them then. They were the most intelligent people I knew, so I tried to take their word for it, though I kept up with Bible reading because the claim that it was unnecessary never sat well. I was praying constantly for God's protection, even when it meant I had to hide in the bathroom to do it so people wouldn't obtain further ammo for their "Miya's losing it" case. The fear slowly started easing up.

When I joined the Bible study group at school, it was pointed out to me during a discussion that Hell and demons do exist, as seen throughout Scripture. I couldn't argue.

*But my family said . . . So wait . . . Does this mean I need to be scared again?*

I don't believe in cherry-picking the Bible. I believe we need to either accept or reject the whole thing. Obviously, that doesn't mean we have to understand every single thing, that different interpretations can't exist, or that we're not allowed to wrestle with things. That's all inevitable. But if we choose to believe in Jesus and accept the parts of Scripture that we like, I don't believe that we can write off the more confusing and uncomfortable parts as false.

What I would come to learn later and what no one ever told me growing up is that Jesus gives us authority over the enemy and his lackeys. Through Christ, we have the power to cast those things out and make them flee. The Spirit of God lives in us if we give our hearts to Him.

> When the seventy-two disciples returned, they joyfully reported to him, "Lord, even the demons obey us when we use your name!" "Yes," he told them, "I saw Satan fall from heaven like lightning! Look, I have given you authority over all the power of the enemy, and you can walk among snakes and scorpions and crush them. Nothing will injure you. But don't rejoice because evil spirits obey you; rejoice because your names are registered in heaven" (Luke 10:17-19).

Disregard all those lies in Hollywood, where the characters can supposedly do nothing but helplessly run away, only to inevitably be caught in the end, no matter what. If we have the Holy Spirit, we have power in the name of Jesus as His followers. I wish someone would have told me all of this sooner, before this ordeal shaved years off my life.

Looking back, do I think there was actually a single demon following me everywhere and trying to take over my body like in that movie? Probably not. Do I believe I was being spiritually tormented by the enemy through fear? Absolutely. To this day, I still stay away from creepy things, whether horror movies or otherwise, because I know how sadistic my anxiety is and how easily it gets set off. I'd much rather focus on rejoicing that my name is written in Heaven.

As we're encouraged in Philippians 4:8, "And now, dear brothers and sisters, one final thing. Fix your thoughts on what is true, and honorable, and right, and pure, and lovely, and admirable. Think about things that are excellent and worthy of praise." Different people have different limits and triggers (or a lack thereof), and that's okay. This helped me learn the importance of personal boundaries and discernment. The enemy does not get the final say over us. We are safe in Christ.

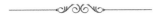

Waking up one day to find strange rashes randomly spread all over my body was a recipe for another deliciously disastrous treat that my anxiety monster happily devoured. They were oddly shaped and would appear every time I scratched my skin or applied pressure. It seriously looked like a disturbing, contagious infection that I probably needed to be hospitalized for—or, at least, quarantined—like those gross, graphic images you see in biology textbooks. It's not fun to suddenly see that stuff on your own body.

Days later, other weird symptoms were rolling in even before the panic did. Ongoing fevers ended up lasting for months. All my limbs randomly went numb—the tingly sensation sometimes shooting rapidly through them like needles. Consistent nausea accompanied the sensation of a cactus in my throat and agonizing pain in my joints, as if I'd aged fifty years overnight. I lost feeling in my back on occasion.

I went to several doctors in multiple cities. No one knew what was going on. Many of them brushed it off as nothing and said that I was probably just stressed and being dramatic. It was disheartening to learn that a lot of doctors don't seem to care in the slightest about their patients. Every visit basically went like this:

"I don't know what's wrong with you. Yes, I see the physical marks on your skin as evidence that something's going on, but it's still just in your head. At the same time, you'll probably have this incurable pain for the rest of your life. It'll also keep getting worse. Bummer. Go home and take a painkiller, I guess. Now, pay up and get out."

The visits were often followed by encouraging pep talks from family members. "Shut up about your health already! It's all in your head! There's absolutely nothing going on with your body. You need counseling to get rid of all your crazy."

I obeyed my family's orders and went to a counselor for a while. This person was supposed to tell me I was imagining it all and explain how to turn it off. Instead, I was told, "If you're running fevers, something *is* wrong with you medically. I can try to help a little with the anxiety, but you need to see a medical doctor."

I'm pretty sure this qualified me as a candidate for obtaining the "Running Around in Circles" award of the year. There were definitely some anxiety-induced symptoms on top of everything else, to be fair. That season was also when I learned the hard way to never Google my symptoms.

I clung to God and prayed so much and so hard. I begged for healing. I pleaded for Him to not let me become paralyzed, or die from Lyme disease, or develop cancer, or any other scary thing that Dr. Internet said would likely be my fate for which I should just start planning my funeral. I was hesitant to fall asleep most nights, with the looming fear that I might not wake up or would arise with a bunch of new, painful, terrifying symptoms. How much worse would this pain be in thirty years if it really was going to stay forever?

To quote an actual journal entry from that time:

> God, I NEED YOU. I need Your healing SO badly. Will I ever get better? What is Your will? Your plan for my life? Is it Your will that I remain sick, or that I get arthritis this young? That I live with the pain? I pray that happens ONLY if it is truly Your will. If not . . . Lord, please PLEASE heal me. Protect me from further damage. Make me well again. My life is in Your hands. You gave it to me in the first place, after all.

Eventually I went to an allergist, even though by then, I was pretty sure it wasn't allergies I was dealing with. But it was there that I finally got some peace of mind.

"Oh yeah, we see people with your condition come in all the time. It's a viral infection, but it's nothing serious, and it won't last forever. It usually just takes several months to go away. You can take medicine to ease the symptoms, but I promise it'll go away."

Many unnecessary medical bills later, I finally had an answer. It did indeed go away, and my gratitude was immense.

This was another instance where I believe the enemy was tormenting me with fear. I honestly can't imagine having anxiety to the level that I do and going through terrifying situations without knowing God. Even when I'm scared to death about something or nothing, I always have a loving Father to cling to and hope in. What a privilege that is.

Fear is such a liar. The Bible tells us not to be afraid, and I think we all know how hard that can be, especially those of us with inner anxiety monsters that refuse to pipe down and take a day off. I absolutely support things like medication, deep breathing, therapy, and other strategies to help combat anxiety. I partake in these things regularly. For the Christian, I also think a massively important thing is what I've been shown through experience: hold on to God through it all, in all of our imperfect ways.

Hold on until our knuckles are white and our nails have dug in. Hold on to the One Who holds the universe with whatever strength we can muster. This is far easier said than done—but always worth the fight.

# CHAPTER TEN
## *Adventures with God*

I originally didn't want to go to college. I wasn't ready yet. I'd be on my own in a different town with no familiar faces. While nothing could persuade me to continue living in an actual toaster oven, barring a Divine command from God, I still didn't want to leave my friends and cats behind. During that time, there was actually a fair amount of peace at home. It was as if I was being pulled away from my life by the roots when all was finally well.

Uncertainty has always been daunting. I didn't have the first clue on what to expect from the scary prospect of adulting. Any vague preconceptions I had were negative. People thought it was appropriate to share ever-so-delightful scenarios with me, beginning in early childhood and continuing for as long as I can remember. I was consistently told that college is so unimaginably hard and draining that it would utterly wreck me from the inside out. Aside from the apparent soul-crushing studies, it would be all about wild parties, with shady characters everywhere and dangerous things happening on the regular. But I'd still be required to be a party animal whether or not I wanted to because it's the law. At the same time, I wouldn't be able to sleep, bathe, or do anything ever because schoolwork would consume every second of my days. Also, I'd probably starve to death because everyone knows college students have empty bank accounts. If I dared to step foot outside at night, I'd get mugged or something. I wouldn't have any space to breathe in my dorm. Professors have zero mercy and would hate me unless I was perfect. My problems would all be my own, and no one would ever care or help.

This is why I always found it odd when people asked why I wasn't excited to start this new chapter. Regardless, I knew God had my back, and we'd get through this just like everything else.

I somehow missed the memo that the school had given me my new email in advance, so I wasn't able to connect with my future roommates or have any idea who they were until I got there. Naturally, my mind was fixed on the possibility of my life turning into a horror movie, since there was no telling what kind of people they would be. Would I get stabbed in my sleep? You never know, right? It happens, I'd heard.

Great news, though—I did not get serial killer roommates or become the star of a gloomy news headline. It was truly amazing, in all seriousness. The three of us became extremely close and had a lot of fun, despite us all being so different. We would spend night after night watching old cartoons, creating art or coloring in our cutesy coloring books, laughing at goofy videos, and chatting about life happenings. We became a little family, and I loved them dearly.

The biggest shocker from college, however, was the magical thing that happened within me.

Miya: "Guess what, world?! I'm an extrovert now!"

The world, probably: "When is the apocalypse? Tomorrow? Next week?"

It wasn't long before my introversion and anything resembling shyness fled from battle. To this day, I don't know how that happened, though I'd venture to guess it had something to do with the way the first week's events set the stage.

I was still naturally a bit timid at first and remained a hermit in my dorm, not really knowing my way around campus yet, much less the town, which may or may not have been safe. The stranger-danger stuff that was hammered into my skull all my life was still low-key scaring me as an adult. I wasn't really in the mood to get attacked or kidnapped by a creep during my first week of college.

The weekend before classes started, I ended up going to some random bonfire at the last minute, mainly so I could say I did at least one social thing. I had zero interest or intention of getting into the party scene, so this event sounded safe. I thought it was just going to be a regular, uneventful type of gathering. The plan was to stand around, make forced small talk with a couple people, eat snacks, and retreat back to safety. Then I found out it was hosted by the massive, yet welcoming campus ministry group, InterVarsity. Knowing that changed everything.

It was a full "house" in the parking lot behind the student union that evening. Small circles of people covered the area. I awkwardly walked up to one of those circles and started saying stuff, trying not to look completely clueless and hoping for the best. Color me surprised when the awkwardness vanished immediately. They welcomed me with open arms as I interrupted their conversation and began introducing me to several seasoned members. It was as if I was already one of them. I received countless phone numbers from all these new friends before we even left the parking lot. I wasn't eagerly looking for opportunities to jump ship and flee back to safety.

We all headed out to a forest for the bonfire, where I befriended more people while trying to decipher faces from the sole light source of the flames. One leader invited me to tag along with her and her roommates to get food and watch a movie at their place after the event. Not once did I feel intrusive or begrudgingly tolerated by any of them.

Despite that awesome night, I didn't intend to actually join the group. Leaders would text me during the weeks to come, inviting me to their Thursday night service, known as "Large Group." I kept blowing it off, as I was already planning to join a Lutheran group that I'd reached out to beforehand. There was no need for another campus ministry.

But then guilt got the best of me. I figured it couldn't hurt to at least try it, even if it was just because I felt bad for ignoring the invites. Just once. That's it.

Walking up the steps to the social sciences building that night, I ran into a familiar face from the Lutheran group and was immediately introduced to her circle. Like the bonfire, I was almost effortlessly befriending people left and right. There were hundreds of people there, but I didn't feel overwhelmed. It was exciting somehow, like discovering Narnia for the first time but without an evil witch killing the mood. I couldn't get enough.

I still don't know how my autistic brain wasn't overwhelmed even a little by any of this. But given the fact that I was talking to people and being social, no longer that outcast hiding in the corner, I believed more strongly than ever that I wasn't autistic anymore. And yes, I was unknowingly mega-masking and very much kidding myself.

The Large Group service was like nothing I'd ever experienced. I took a seat with my new buddies in the large auditorium, where red curtains served as a fancy backdrop for the band and speaker on stage. Fittingly, the message was about hospitality and welcoming strangers.

"We shouldn't be inhospitable toward those who are different from us," the speaker said.

She was talking more about different ethnic cultures, but I couldn't help but feel that personally. I was always viewed as *different*, to some extent, by the world—and usually not in a positive way. The hospitality I was being shown by the group was a strong indication that they took that goal seriously. I loved how she took her time and had so much heart behind her message, not just going through the motions.

Not to sound overly dramatic, but during worship, I felt my spirit come alive in a way I don't think I ever had until then. People were visibly passionate, excited to worship their Creator. Nearly everyone had their hands in the air. Some were on their knees, singing at the top of their lungs, almost louder than the band. They were undignified and unashamed. It was a beautiful thing that I'd never seen before, and I felt such freedom seeing that it's actually a thing to be enthusiastic and that I was allowed to get into it.

The band started playing "How He Loves," which was my favorite song to worship to at the time thanks to my favorite band Flyleaf's cover. I raised my arm toward the sky for the first time and got swept away in praise. I felt so alive, proclaiming with my body and soul that I loved God and that He is good. I was one with the family of Heaven. No more persuasion was needed. I knew this was a group I wanted to be in. I never missed a service after that.

After Large Group, we'd always go to a coffee shop or a dorm lounge, talking, laughing, playing billiards games, and hanging out until two in the morning. It was newly extroverted Miya's favorite day of the week.

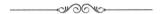

Freedom was no longer a pipe dream. It was such a mind-blowing, refreshing feeling that I never expected—being able to make my own decisions, do what I wanted, and just breathe freely without anyone watching over my shoulder. I never imagined I'd be able to have that kind of life. Even simple things like going to the cafeteria would have me saying to myself, "How cool is it that I get to do this? And on my own, too? I don't need anyone's permission to exist and live life."

"Well, *duh*," I hear you say. "That's the whole reason people get excited to go to college and be on their own. Everyone knows that." You'd think. I guess there was one positive outcome from the horror stories I was given growing up. With such low expectations, I was delightfully surprised and relieved when I actually got there. Feeling unchained and in control of my life, even in the small things, was one of the most welcome surprises ever to come my way. Independence played a part, but it was healthy and life-giving community that truly strengthened my relationship with God.

One afternoon during the first week of school, I was walking down the pedway where different clubs were always advertising themselves. I ignored them. And then I stopped at one for no particular reason. It was for Campus Crusade (Cru). I didn't want to be rude, so I wrote down my contact information when asked, even though I had no intention of joining yet another church group.

Less than two weeks later, I was a regular attendee of their women's small group. Stopping at a seemingly random booth that day must've been a Divine appointment. I made some lovely friends there, as well—one of whom would become my roommate for several years, starting with a life-saving incident that would occur soon after.

Some months later, I was also attending Cru's main worship service, campus outreach, and various volunteer events. I wanted to be involved in *everything,* going to all three campus ministry groups every single week to learn more about God and be with my pals. It was all fuel for my soul in every sense. I'd frequently just sit in the student union or some other public place because chances are I'd run into someone I knew, and we'd hang out right then and there. I didn't want to just be home by myself because that was so much less exciting.

One of the most valuable things I learned in college was the significance of exploring different churches and doctrines—with discernment, of course—instead of stubbornly sticking to the only thing I'd ever known. As time went on, I realized I didn't really identify with the denomination of my youth anymore. I was just a plain ol' Christian who loved the Lord and wanted to seek Him.

Toward the end of the year, I was urged by multiple people to choose one of the groups I was in. They said I should commit to one, instead of always running back and forth and trying to do *all* the things. I was immediately offended.

What was wrong with being so involved? Why would they criticize me for being social? Didn't they know how big of a deal that was for me?

After being advised more than once, I took time to really think about it and begrudgingly admitted they were right. I was thinking of becoming a leader at some point, after all—another big thing to sign up for, proving that I was social and competent and definitely not shy! The following year, I settled on InterVarsity.

I was still inexplicably extroverted over the next few years and extremely proud of myself. I became a small group co-leader for a short time, after endless encouragement from my lovely mentor at the time, Gloria. She was an awesome influence I honestly believe was at least part of the reason why I became so extroverted and confident (more autistic mimicking, unbeknownst to me at the time). I was dealing with a lot of drama and heartbreak that year, but she was with me through it all.

Reality ended in disappointment compared to the idea. Even though I was sure I wanted to become a leader, my heart wasn't in it when the time came. Preparing lessons felt way more like a chore than a passion. I felt out of my element because the members of my small group were all way smarter than me. What right did I, an absolute simpleton, have leading them? I know that's not necessarily a good reason, but it's how I often feel in these situations. I was just glad I wasn't leading it alone. Most of the time I was just there, letting the others do the talking. Regardless of the situation or what it was for, I've never felt like leader material. That's usually seen as a terrible thing by our culture, but I wonder about that sometimes. There's great value in being a regular team member as well.

Sadly, the time came at the beginning of year three for me to say goodbye to InterVarsity, despite how much I had loved it for a season. Things were changing, and fears of becoming an outcast again were creeping up. So I fled. Wanting to start fresh, I knew there was one group remaining that seemed popular and legit—Chi Alpha (fun fact: not a sorority or fraternity).

I had asked a friend to come with me the first couple of times, in case there were any red flags. But what I experienced was the most genuinely loving and welcoming community I had ever been to, even after InterVarsity had set the bar high.

Walking into the little blue building at the edge of campus that night, it was as if people were eagerly waiting to meet us and introduce themselves. One after another, people came to say hello. It wasn't just obligatory, forced small talk. I could tell that they were genuinely interested in getting to know me and viewed me as a valuable sister in Christ, not just another body in the building.

Everything I had loved about InterVarsity was there, though the group was much smaller. My cautious self sat there listening to the sermon, intently waiting to hear any kind of shady theology. There wasn't any.

It turned out that a handful of people I already knew were in the group. I had met one girl previously, who ended up becoming my small group leader and a dear friend to this day. Violet is a beautiful soul who has such profound wisdom on every level. She had a way of helping me see meanings in Scripture and God's character like I never had before. She always helped me come back to my senses when I was having family problems, work problems, or ridiculous boy problems. She's the kind of person who just naturally blesses anyone she comes into contact with.

After Bible study one night, she informed me that the group would be having a story night in place of a sermon and asked if I wanted to share my testimony. She assured me I was allowed to, despite having only been in Chi Alpha for a few weeks. Recalling that day at my home church when I'd shared my story and all the inspiration that followed, I jumped at the opportunity.

Like the last time, a shocking number of people came to talk to me afterward and said my story was inspiring. I think it would be cool if this were a more common practice in churches—letting people share their stories, even if they're not in leadership positions. I befriended so many more people after that, which might not have happened otherwise. I felt seen and understood.

Chi Alpha became my home, both figuratively and literally. They let me live in their building for a month during a school break when I was banished from my family's house and had nowhere else to go. I stayed in the group for over four years; graduation didn't stop me. It's where I met my husband. It's where I finally came to a place of feeling safe enough to be vulnerable about my struggles. I learned so much from this found family.

I'm realizing more and more over time how immensely important community is. Of course, it was much easier for me back in those days. I was able to mask extremely well, even if I didn't acknowledge I was doing so due to the freedom high and ignorance. Nowadays, as an introverted misfit who can no longer mask to that degree, I know full well how difficult the community aspect can be for many. To be clear, no one should feel shame about things like spotty church attendance or struggling in any way with a social life. Sometimes, I need a break. Life happens. Mental health struggles happen. But I've noticed that when I make a habit of playing hooky from church and actively avoiding human contact, I start to feel the negative effects. I have less accountability.

We were made to be in some sort of community. This is especially true for the Christian, I think. Even the most introverted introverts need other people in their lives in some capacity.

# CHAPTER ELEVEN
## Desperate Times

A lot of change was happening back at home—the worst and most unpredictable kind. Once again, people I had placed my trust in were betraying it in their own unique ways. I theorize that much of this particular switch had to do with the fact that yet another stepfamily had entered the scene, and I didn't appear impressive enough to meet their standards.

Being away at college, even just for a semester, made me feel so much more grown up, and I was stoked to be treated with dignity and respect upon returning home. They would see that I had a lot of new appreciation for life and was slowly but surely learning how to take care of myself and navigate the world. They'd learn that I had made many wonderful friends, was volunteering for various events, and was doing extremely well in classes—all with a faith stronger than ever and the highest level of happiness to date. Surely, this all meant I was worthy of respect and being treated like a human being.

Except none of that mattered in the slightest. As it transpired, all my family cared about was the fact that I hadn't been able to land a part-time job yet. I wasn't neglecting it. The competition was, to put it lightly, completely insane. Regardless of effort, I was seen as worthless trash without a job, even though I had some financial aid and my family wasn't exactly experiencing financial hardship, so having a little extra income wasn't urgent. But I discovered there was a hard line in determining whether I was valid as a human being or the scum of the earth. I didn't know this line existed. I assumed they hired contractors to install it while I was away because it definitely wasn't there before.

I wanted to go on a church trip over spring break, but that desire proved to be outrageous and should not have been brought up. If I'd had time travel powers back then, I would've gone back and erased the moment I asked for permission, possibly preventing the explosion to end all explosions. Then again, that still wouldn't have guaranteed safety.

You might be wondering, "Why on earth haven't you cut these people off at this point?" The short answer is that it's complicated. Maybe just imagine a masterfully constructed combination of brainwashing and emotional manipulation, financial dependence, and general familial obligation, knowing they used to be nicer, along with the fact that I had believed that loving my neighbor and forgiving people meant gritting my teeth and bearing abuse endlessly, with no accountability. And for whatever reason, part of me still wanted their approval.

In the spirit of anonymity, this family member will henceforth be referred to as The Dictator. Keeping my head up and remaining optimistic that things would get better, I got home after visiting some relatives one night and was met with The Dictator's long, vicious burst of rage. They directed me to a bedroom, along with some siblings as an audience, and screamed at me at the top of their lungs for what felt like hours. It wasn't just a short-lived tantrum like usual. The threats remained in place, even after they calmed down. This person always yelled a lot and was regularly angry. But this was something else.

The summary:

1.  I didn't deserve to be in college anymore, since I was so irresponsible.

2.  I was nothing more than a lazy, disrespectful, good-for-nothing disgrace to the family. My inability to find a job within the first few months of school was equivalent to a lack of gratitude and respect.

3. I'd contributed nothing to the family outside of bringing hardship and misery upon them, forcing them through the pain of providing basic needs like food and shelter since the day I was born. I should be praising them for not letting me starve to death as a child.

4. They wanted to test a sample of my hair for drugs.

I wish I could say this melodramatic-sounding list is in any way an exaggeration.

Now that I was a legal adult, it was time for them to *really* crack down. I was threatened to have everything taken away, as The Dictator still had that kind of authority and exploited my financial dependence for control. They were the boss, and I wasn't allowed to have a voice. I was going to be pulled out of school with all funding cut off and would either need to be a perfect, obedient robot living under constant supervision, or would be kicked out and likely end up on the streets. Or I would be sleeping on a friend's couch and being a burden, which I'd feel too guilty about.

I received constant reminders that running to other family members for help wasn't an option because, of course, they're all evil and couldn't be trusted and didn't actually care about me.

When I look back, I think that underneath all the yelling and fury was deep-rooted, ableist disappointment that I wasn't passing as neurotypical as flawlessly as they wanted. I should've been able to easily interview for jobs and make them love me and my personality. I should've been able to act just like the new step-siblings. At the end of the day, I became the designated scapegoat once more. At least this time around, I had my Jesus to cling to. But even with my faith, there appeared to be no way out of this mess.

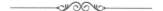

I'd never lived in a cold climate before college. Every snowstorm filled me with gratitude that I had shelter but also broke my heart to think about how some people had to sleep outside. Many people saw my dorm room as a tiny box with three poor souls crammed in it. To me, it was home. It was a safe place that I was lucky to have. I loved that box.

As sad of a reality as it is, I got more exposure to homelessness in my college town than ever before. I so badly wished I could help. When I thought about the very real possibility that I might wind up losing everything and sleeping in the snow, my panic meter skyrocketed like never before. Hypothetical *what if* scenarios didn't compare to something that was likely going to happen if all else failed.

I was given a deadline to find a job, with the new requirement being upped to full-time employment by May 13. If I missed it, I was toast. I was hoping that if I kissed up to The Dictator like my life depended on it—and it did—and found something in my college town, maybe I'd be shown mercy and would get to stay in school after all. Despite The Dictator's assurance that I was finished and they wouldn't reconsider, I'd learned a few survival strategies in the art of kissing up throughout the years: give them lots of praise, smile constantly, always appear visibly productive and report my progress in detail at the end of each day, and say thank you for literally everything at every moment, including insults and abuse. So I switched into high gear. Online job applications and occasional in-person visits weren't enough anymore. Every single day, I dressed up in the fanciest clothing I owned, walked all around town until my pretty shoes were stained with blood, and applied for a position at nearly every business in sight—even if I had no idea who they were or what they did. I put on a happy face as if I wasn't scared out of my mind because most companies probably don't want to hire some crazy lady who comes in bawling and begging them to save her life. I would call them all to follow up and irritate them every day, absolutely desperate that someone would have compassion and hire me.

*I don't care what position. Just give me* something. *I'll scrub floors with a toothbrush if that's what you want.*

There was also the issue of finding a place to live for the summer, even though I still didn't know the town very well and didn't have transportation. As a freshman who wasn't very far into adulting, I didn't yet understand the processes involved in leasing. I didn't know anyone who was staying in town over the summer and also needed a roommate, though it wouldn't matter either way, considering the astronomical housing costs that the town is infamous for. Regardless, I desperately continued applying for jobs in hopes that maybe something miraculous would happen because God is far bigger than any ridiculous circumstance. I sent cheesy thank you cards to all the managers just for taking my application and then another for interviewing me, hoping it might set me apart. I was cringing at the fakeness and absurdity of it all.

Unfortunately, my vigorous efforts didn't matter. It was nearly impossible to find a job as a full-time student in an overcrowded town to begin with, but once customer service managers heard my naturally quiet voice and speech impediment, the answer was always no. It wasn't a lack of effort or professionalism but my voice that was the problem, as some of them informed me. The thank you cards were a nice gesture, but that didn't make them want me as an employee representing, or embarrassing, their company. They had hundreds upon hundreds of other applicants who were loud and didn't have speech impediments.

Panic attacks became an almost daily occurrence. Unable to concentrate in class, I would often leave so I could lock myself in a bathroom stall and cry, hyperventilate, and call all of the businesses for the umpteenth time to see if there was any hope. All I got was the same annoyed script: "We'll call you someday if we're interested."

*"Someday" doesn't work for me. I can already feel the shackles forming around my ankles. But thanks.*

Throughout all this madness, I continued to cling to God, praying ceaselessly, begging for provision. I wanted to trust in Him so badly, but the panic was too much sometimes. But I knew that whatever happened or didn't happen, He was good and would be with me through everything. Even if I lost everything else, I would still have Him. It took all the childlike faith I could muster, trying to trust that my True Parent would take care of me one way or another.

Almost at my limit, I figured the only realistic thing I could do was say goodbye to every ounce of freedom I had. I could still hear The Dictator's voice, telling me it's not working out because I'm not trying hard enough and that it should be simple. The act of trying wasn't good enough, but I still needed to try harder. I needed to feel guilty after all they'd sacrificed to raise the useless, lazy trash that I was. I didn't deserve to exist in this world because I wasn't contributing enough. But of course, I must remember that they tell me all of this because they love me.

I talked through this whole situation with several of my church group leaders. They offered all the love and support they could, feeling sorry that they couldn't do anything to fix a financial predicament of this magnitude. One of them had informed me of a painting position for students at facility services during the earlier stages of my search. I had, of course, applied for that even before the big explosion at home but assumed the familiar crickets meant it wasn't happening nor would it magically change now that I was utterly desperate. The clock was ticking—thirty-four days until the deadline.

I came back to my dorm after a class I was most definitely not present for and opened my laptop for more job searching, shifting to places in my hometown because I was beginning to accept my fate. A new email caught my eye: the campus paint shop manager had reached out with an interview invitation. Huzzah! Except by that point, I fully expected to be rejected yet again and knew it probably wouldn't pay enough for me to be able to live on my own, regardless. But as a last-ditch effort, I went anyway. Thirty-three days were left.

The manager explained that I'd just be painting walls with zero customer service requirements—perfect for my in-denial-but-very-real autism. It sounded ideal, but I still had doubts about how financially realistic this would be. Then came the game-changer.

"And if you work full-time, you'll get free housing for the summer," he said.

"Did you just say *free* housing?" I asked, incredulous. "Did I hear that right? Like, literally free?"

"Yeah, all of our full-timers get free housing during those months if they want it."

"But I'll have to pay it back later, right?"

"Nope. No strings attached besides working full-time. You'll get to live in the new, fully furnished apartments on campus."

My soaring hope started arm-wrestling with my paranoia. "Completely free? For real? There's gotta be a catch . . . "

"Just don't get fired, obviously, and you'll be good. You won't get fired unless you really do something terrible."

"When is the start date?"

"May 13."

I was hired on the spot. I would start on the exact day that I needed to. I wouldn't need to pay a dime for rent that summer. It felt way too good to be true. Reading that scenario in a book probably makes it sound extra questionable. You may be wondering how the scam was revealed or what went wrong. Sorry to be anticlimactic, but it was legit. There was no catch, and I did not get fired. God graciously provided literally exactly what I needed, and because of this, I was able to continue going to school.

I found all of this out right after my time slot to enroll in housing for the following school year had closed—yet another problem to deal with but God had my back. I was talking about it with my friend Hannah during Bible study when she said she was looking for a roommate for the next school year. She explained that she could pull me with her and would take care of the logistics. Another crisis averted at the last minute. We became roommates for the next four years.

God really heard me all those times I cried out to Him. Dropping out of college and living like a chained-up hostage forever weren't on His agenda for me. Naturally, the threats, gaslighting, and other controlling behaviors from The Dictator didn't stop, despite the temporary appeasement. But God never let me fall. I always try to remember things like this whenever I'm afraid. He has always taken care of me, and He always will.

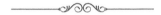

My infamous anxiety monster was acting up around the start date of the job. I'd expect no less from the punk—stomping on the ground, scratching at the walls, breaking things like he owns the place, and reminding me of what I was told my whole life: how working is the worst thing ever, how much I'll hate life, how I need to be perfect at all times, and how outrageously draining it would be.

"Perhaps you're safe for *now*," he taunted, "but for how long? Landing a job was the easy part. What makes you think you can handle the *real* challenge—keeping it?"

"Hmm. You have a point. After all . . . "

*What if I mess up and get fired, losing my housing in the process? What if no one likes me there? What if I get seriously injured? What if I get hit on by creepy men? What if I just can't handle it? What if . . .*

I had an inevitable breakdown the day before I had to move out of my dorm, after my roommates left and everything started becoming real. Work would be starting the day after I transferred into the new place. Everything was changing so rapidly. Change tends to be difficult for autistics.

When the scary day came, I headed out at the crack of dawn, arrived at the paint shop embarrassingly early because I'd been told that's a good look, sat there awkwardly for an eternity before the others arrived, and prayed that I wouldn't fail.

We all headed into the meeting room, and they assigned everyone to a crew. I was skipped.

*Oh no. Please don't let this be an indicator of catastrophe. Did my paperwork get lost? Was I not actually hired? Did they change their minds at the last second? I'm gonna lose my new apartment, and I'll have to sell everything I own and try to make it on the streets and—*

Reality: an honest mistake that was fixed in half a second.

Once we got going, it was pretty smooth sailing. Thanks be to God, I ended up loving it there. It was painfully evident and almost laughable to some of the seasoned workers how nervous I was at the beginning, which became a running joke later. I didn't think my body was visibly shaking, but alas. There was a whole story behind my amplified fear that they didn't know about, but there was also a story of protection and answered prayers—a story I hoped I'd get to share someday.

As with anything, there were naturally ups and downs. Some days were awesome, and others had me crawling out of my skin. But at the end of the day, I couldn't be anything but grateful. That job was the whole reason I was able to be there at all. God used it to save me from ruin, and I was overflowing with joy. I'd be painting walls, jamming out to Flyleaf and Skillet, and smiling like a doofus because I loved God and was so thankful to be there, alive.

God gave me a heart for all the people there, and I wound up loving them all dearly—even the ones who weren't always nice. I made many wonderful friends, some of whom I'm still close with to this day. It was admittedly a bit of a culture shock at first, since this group was so different from the crowd I was used to running with. I was the only Christian for a while, but it was a good and needed experience to step out of my bubble and get to know people who were different from me. Though we didn't always see eye to eye on everything, we got along very well and had a lot of good times—whether it was loudly singing along to music while we worked, building mattress forts when we had to clear furniture out of rooms, taking goofy selfies, eating food, talking about life, or whatever else. Many of them challenged my beliefs in ways no one ever had before, which inspired me to get deeper into theology. I grew closer to God as a result.

God can use mundane things like painting walls for His glory. He can take desperate times and turn them into something profoundly awesome.

# CHAPTER TWELVE
## Now I'm Supposed to Pursue Romance?

"Ugh, when are you *ever* gonna get a boyfriend, Miya? Hurry up already! What's wrong with you?"

I lost count by the time I was a teenager of how many times I heard that. It was yet another supposed life requirement that I was failing to meet. B.C. Miya's mental response was always along the lines of, "Oh, save it! There's no chance a guy would ever be the slightest bit interested in someone like me, anyway. But I don't even care about guys because I hate people. Just drop it already!"

Christian Miya's mental response was, "Whoa, whoa! Hold on! I'm just now learning how to make *friends*. One thing at a time!"

Romance was not at all on my radar until the last couple months of high school when I had my first real crush, with an actual interest in dating instead of just, "Oh, sure, I guess he's cute. Whatever." It didn't happen, by the way. The whole thing was very awkward. My memory is foggy on most of the details, and frankly, I'd like to keep it that way.

I could never understand what the big deal was when my friends talked about their crushes or why almost every song I'd ever heard was about romance. It got super annoying. Seriously, what was all the fuss about?

Then more epiphany bowling balls dropped on my head at a random, inexplicable time. College came around, and I felt like a total newbie in this department, thrown into the fire with no training and going through a phase that I should've gone through several years prior: being a boy-crazy, blushing mess all the time and actually wanting to date, even though the idea of it was a little bit terrifying. Interacting with the opposite sex felt almost foreign, as I never really had many male friends. Any time I managed to make a guy friend or two, several individuals would get their hopes up for me and assumed I was finally in love simply because he was a living, breathing human who happened to be male. Were they to look into my head and see what was actually going on, they'd find I was simply proud of myself on a social level for even having guy friends at all, as I was usually intimidated by the male species.

As it would turn out, if I wanted to date, it meant that I actually had to put myself out there and actually talk to guys—regularly—and flirt—whatever that is. This form of rocket science sounded more complicated than my macroeconomics class that made my brain glitch on a daily basis.

Fortunately, much of it wasn't as difficult or scary as I expected. Well, I would never want to watch reruns of my weak, painful attempts at what was supposed to resemble flirting, as I would probably drop dead from cringe overload. It could be a free showing, and I'd still want my money back.

But I tried. It was something. F plus for effort?

The timidity was a strange thing, even for me. I don't know why, but I was always extra wary around guys most of the time, despite growing up with a bunch of boys. Anytime a female friend or family member talked about their potential love interests or the possibility of dating, I couldn't be happy for them, only nervous.

"What if he hurts you? What if he's abusive? How do you know you can trust him?" I'd want to ask.

I don't know where that came from exactly. I can't recall witnessing any domestic violence between partners as a kid—not physically, anyway. There was just a lot of yelling on both sides. Maybe all the scary screaming made me fear that violence would eventually follow. Whatever the reason, the idea of a girl getting with a guy sounded a bit dangerous to me, especially if one dated a beefy, muscular man. I guess I knew a lot of those as a kid, now that I think about it.

I always wanted to say, "Sure, they're all nice, non-violent men. But what if something goes wrong, and that changes? As I've been taught, people change their minds all the time."

Evidently, I got over that fear at some point, as I was pursuing romance myself. How that happened was beyond me. The legitimate desire for that type of intimacy with someone intensified, and those reservations flew out the window. After a few letdowns and realizing that most of my guy friends from classes probably weren't in my best interest for several reasons, I finally woke up to what should've been obvious to me in the first place: I needed to find someone who loved Jesus and lived like it—someone who bore spiritual fruit and with whom I could pursue the Lord. Discernment was crucial.

One problem, though—pretty much none of the Christian men I knew were single. The male-to-single-female ratio was disproportionate in all the groups I'd been in. My chances of being selected by someone were probably nonexistent.

I tried to keep the whole thing lighthearted and not worry about dating too much. Life was still good in other ways, with so much to be thankful for. I had some friends at the time who were frequently in bad moods and complaining about their singleness. I was hardcore judging them.

*I would* never *throw tantrums over being single!*

A month later, I was throwing tantrums over being single.

What was supposed to be lighthearted turned into obsessing over being "forever alone." Believing that I was no longer autistic and having worked hard to forsake many of my allegedly less desirable qualities (like being quiet), still feeling unwanted really stung. I entered a couple of pretty intense—albeit relatively short—on-and-off seasons of extreme self-loathing for that reason. I knew my worth didn't depend on having a significant other, but it was the principle of it. Being wanted by no one made it extremely difficult not to believe something was wrong with me, and that in itself was triggering.

I took one of those online quizzes on what kind of person I'm meant to be with based on my personality. My result: a robot programmed to love. Normally, I'd appreciate the comedy, but this wasn't the best time.

There would be darker times and episodes of torment, where I'd be breaking my back trying to stop thinking about it because that would be the healthy and logical thing to do. Funny how attempting to forcefully stop thinking about any particular thing tends to have the opposite effect.

I still remember my darkened dorm room matching my dark mood. I'd bury myself under the blankets to block out the single source of light seeping through the edges of the blinds. The ringing silence enveloped me, save for the occasional footsteps in the hallway. My mind would rapidly spiral, falling off the highest ledge and smacking down on the pavement like Chutes and Ladders, except I missed the slide.

I truly believed I'd never be worth anyone's time or affection. I was stuck in an infinite Möbius strip of being rejected because I couldn't seem to fully discard every last ounce of lingering awkwardness.

*It's almost as if I'm still autis—*

Nope. I couldn't go there. I shoved the idea back into my mind's dungeon and opted to listen to the enemy's taunts instead.

*It's over. Look what you've done. It could've worked out if you weren't so . . . you. Why can't you just be fully normal and competent, you pathetic embarrassment to the human race? How are you even surprised that no one wants you? You may as well just disappear.*

*When are you* ever *gonna get a boyfriend, Miya? Hurry up already! What's wrong with you?*

The wisest course of action seemed to be mentally gutting myself for being so "old," at the ripe old age of nineteen, and still single with no dating experience because it was obviously my fault. I was letting the onlookers down. I'd also beat myself up for being overly dramatic about the whole thing. There was no winning.

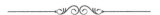

I give this disclaimer half-jokingly because, though I have only positive things to say about my husband, we decided it would be wise to change his name to further protect the identities of others. I asked him what he wanted his fake name to be. He said Akechi, based on his favorite video game character. We're going with it.

Despite the temporary episodes of singleness despair, I was still joyful, living my best life and always praising the Lord. Time went on, and I allowed myself to exhale, leaving the prospect of dating alone and choosing to be thankful for the beautiful life I had.

Come junior year, about a month after joining Chi Alpha, the group was preparing for a Halloween prayer outreach event one night and needed to do some role playing for practice. I volunteered to go up for a round because they all needed to see how brave and not shy I was.

I sat in front of three others, two of whom I'd already met at services. As part of the role play, we went around and "introduced" ourselves to each other.

I turned to the guy on my left, who said, "Hi, I'm Akechi. Nice to meet you. No, really, it's nice to meet you since I actually haven't met you before."

*Oh . . . hey . . . you're cute. Heh. Why haven't I seen you here before? No, stop being weird, Miya. You don't know this guy. Focus on the role play!*

"Hi, I'm Miya. Good to be here."

*But if he's a student leader with this ministry, that means he's a devout Christian seeking after Jesus, right? No, seriously, cut it out. That's not why you're here.*

We completed the practice round and went on with our lives; nothing significant happening. But as the Lord would have it, after that day, we started hanging out on the regular, starting with a mutual interest of playing *Super Smash Bros.* He was far better than me at that game.

I had to put myself out there and initiate much of it, but I figured it was always good to be social. That was my excuse, anyway. Crush or not, I was still Miya, the definitely-not-shy-person. Everyone needed to know it.

The first time we really bonded was during the first Chi Alpha service after winter break. A week prior, my good friend and then-coworker had been teaching me how to do heavy metal screamo. It was one of my top bucket list items because it's hardcore and seemed like a therapeutic way to vent intense emotions. Once an edgy person, always an edgy person (is that how the saying goes?). She had me start off practicing the heavy sighs from the gut while recording the audio on my phone. I experimented with this for a couple hours. A couple of supervisors were very confused when they walked in on us painting and screaming.

I got the basic technique down and was stoked to be able to just make the sound, even though I couldn't make words out of it yet. But I was doing it! I was officially metal!

That night at Chi Alpha was the first of what would be many karaoke sessions after service. It was pretty popular, as a bunch of people signed up and stayed late to watch. I was still recovering from the aftermath of a pretty rough cold, and my throat was still sore. So what did I do to soothe it? A belting screamo performance, of course.

This wave of adrenaline came over me, making it feel urgent and necessary. I thought I'd look awesome and hardcore in front of Akechi, despite not knowing what I was doing. I'd probably sound like a clown doing a terrible impression of a growling tiger, but it still sounded like a good idea. My wonderful friend Taylor agreed to do it with me, since she can actually sing—unlike me, who would shatter every window in that building with my attempts. My screamo is ironically a more pleasant sound.

We decided on "I'm So Sick" by Flyleaf. We practiced in the parking lot before our turn, as she was trying to learn the song altogether. I was still struggling to make out words and phrases through screaming, startling the occasional passerby when I tried. But then it was time. While up there, it somehow came to me. I was making words! I suppose the pressure of a live audience can do the trick in a pinch. Of course, I burst out laughing mid-performance, along with everyone else, because the scream was so unexpected. Akechi got a kick out of the whole thing. My mission was a success. Shortly after, he and I were up there performing the "Pokérap"—instant best friends.

In the many days to follow, we continued bonding as nerd buddies. I never felt stupid or weird to any degree in his presence. That was a pretty rare thing, even in my outgoing, extroverted days. The silly crush became something much more serious. I got to see what an incredible person he is in every way— his love for God, unquestionably genuine kindness toward everyone, profound wisdom, and wholesome sense of humor. He never failed to amaze me.

I repeatedly raised my hopes, only to kick myself for it later. We were just friends. Nothing was going to happen, since he obviously deserved someone better. There were no signs indicating interest. I had failed once again—friend zoned for life.

*Figures. Why would someone as awesome as he is choose me when there are tons of other nice, single girls in Chi Alpha? Ones who are smarter, funnier, prettier, and more interesting and who don't have speech impediments? What in the world was I thinking when I felt I had a chance?*

The enemy of my soul clearly had a jolly good time with my insecurities in that season. The punk really went to town. But then the day came.

Akechi was walking me home after service, since it had gotten dark. After twenty minutes of my incessant info-dumping about the latest anime fan theories I'd learned, we got to the railing outside my dorm, where he paused to say, "So, I think we should talk about what this is and what's going on with us. I'm nervous to say it, but . . . I have feelings for you."

*Wait. Hold up.*

"I wanted to let you know that I do intend to pursue you," he continued, "but I want to take it slow. I'm so glad we got to become good friends first."

*Are you sure you've got the right person?*

I was an ecstatic mess on the inside but kept it together. I think. It was official. We were on the same page. For the first time in my entire life, it wasn't one-sided. This was happening—outside of my head. That night was when we became "unofficially official" (dating without the titles). It would be a little longer before the "unofficial" part dropped.

Junior year ended, and I was working a summer paint shop shift. A mutual friend who was working there handed me a note from Akechi. It was a map for an egg hunt. The previous month, I had been forced to go to my hometown against my will for Easter when I would've much rather stayed for Chi Alpha's event, which included an egg hunt. Since I couldn't go to that one, Akechi planned one himself on campus for me, where he would be waiting at the final egg. I spent the rest of the day wondering how this guy could possibly be so top-tier.

Stoked as I was, I looked down at my gross work outfit covered in paint. I hadn't brought a change of clothes. He wouldn't have cared either way, which was awesome, but I wasn't about to go on my first date ever looking like a doofus who just got destroyed in a mud-colored paintball fight. I quite literally ran all the way home during lunch to get some clothing that made me look human. The personified Sloppy Joe look would have to wait for another day.

Work ended, and I was off on my mission. Eggs were hidden in trees, under cinder blocks, and behind signs and brick walls. Each one had a heartfelt note with a glorious pun related to the candy that was inside.

I had a hard time fathoming the fact that I, of all people, could mean so much to another person. I was just a walking awkward blob, but he evidently didn't see me that way.

The last egg had a longer, more serious note that ended with a question. "Will you take me as your boyfriend?"

I wanted to cry. There have been very few times in life where I felt genuinely treasured. He came out of hiding, and we went on our first real date: enchiladas, a spontaneous movie, and some nerdy anime.

I was almost a senior in college when I went on my first date ever. I was going out with my perfect match, free to be myself every waking moment.

God had provided for me again, even though I had spent years leading up to that point complaining and being melodramatic.

I fell ill for the rest of that summer, shortly after we got together—because of course, I did. It was that intense, unsolvable affliction I described a few chapters ago. But Akechi took care of me whenever he could. He didn't grow impatient. He got to see literal grosser sides of me early on and wasn't repelled.

To think that I beat myself down so much and thought I wouldn't stand a chance in the romance realm, even though God is infinitely bigger than any insecurity. To think I considered myself unworthy based on my own standards.

We got married a couple of years later. He helps me grow and be real. I learn from him every day. I've never felt so safe, in every way, with another person.

Some people think it's pathetic and desperate, as I've been told, to marry your first significant other. Good for them, I guess. They can think that if they want. I'm too busy being grateful.

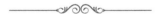

While this is a happy story that happened to work out, I want to be clear. Romance is great, but it's not in any way a requirement for happiness and fulfillment. It certainly doesn't define one's worth. It was infuriating to hear that at one point in my life, especially from people who were in relationships, but it's true (and now I'm the annoying one saying it). It took me experiencing it myself to fully realize it. My worth is no more now than it was when I was single. Romantic partners are not Jesus. Even the kindest, most loving person in the world cannot ultimately fulfill someone.

Attaching self-worth to a romantic partner is such a toxic place to be, and I really don't dig the cultural pressures. I'm still left to wonder, if I never got married but was still the exact same person, how many people would view me as less-than today?

# CHAPTER THIRTEEN
## Here Today

The condo's balcony overlooked the community pool and an abundance of greenery below the cloudy sky. The silence was serene. It was tradition to come to this town with my relatives every summer, though this particular trip sticks out in my mind.

The whole time, I was just overflowing with joy in the Lord and frequently singing praises to Him—probably sounding like a dying animal combined with a garbage disposal, but I didn't care. God still loves it. Adding the fact that He's not a judge at a vocal audition to my list of things to be thankful for, I raised my hands toward the sky out on that patio and felt fully alive.

As someone who occasionally enjoys making visual art, I know how much of a struggle it is to draw things and try to make them look at least somewhat realistic. There are so many nitty-gritty details, and everything is so complex. It takes hours to even make a dent of progress in the overall process. Even when I put in as much effort as I possibly can, my works only come out as mediocre at best. (Probably not even that. I'm not great at the craft.) And yet God paints the real sky every day. Anything we could ever hope to capture in our own works of art is inspired by what He's already made.

I was at the pool later as evening was approaching and the dark clouds were rolling in. The dim lights around the resort flickered gently as wind rustled the trees and soft rain came down. I was in awe at God's handiwork. I happened to catch a single dead leaf in my hand that fell from the tree above. Observing its rusty brown hue and looking back up to the green leaves still connected to the tree, full of life, I was reminded that this life is temporary. It's one of those things we always have in the backs of our minds, but at least in my case, I rarely take the time to really think about it. Ignoring reality doesn't make it go away. Someday, I'm going to be like that crusty, decaying leaf—if I even make it that far. Though I don't have to fear death, I won't be here forever. Tomorrow is never guaranteed. If there was one thing I knew, it was that I wanted my life to be pleasing to my Lord, whatever that may look like. "Our days on earth are like grass; like wildflowers, we bloom and die. The wind blows, and we are gone—as though we had never been here" (Psalm 103:15-16).

Upon returning home, I did a highly unusual thing and spent a day outside. I was lying on a small, grassy hill in front of one of the university's buildings on a very cloudy day. Monsoon season was my favorite, as it was rare to get any kind of precipitation in my hometown. Phoenix residents know how it is. I was watching the misty shapes in the sky move around, catching sight of one forming from nothing and continuing to expand. It was as if God Himself was making the clouds dance, like He knew I'd be watching. Worship music was playing in my headphones as I reflected on my life, full of pure, unadulterated joy.

I wasn't supposed to be there. I was supposed to be back at my family's home living as a suffocating prisoner, with my every move monitored and controlled. Or I was supposed to be stuck outside alone, struggling to survive and about to get caught in the literal storm that was visibly rolling in with nowhere to go. Each day that summer felt hard to believe.

I usually try to avoid thinking about harsh memories, but that doesn't make them any less real. On days like this, though, I couldn't help but feel immense gratitude even when thinking about the most painful times in my life. God rescued me. I cried out to Him over and over, and He pulled me out of the ruins and set me on solid ground. He didn't have to do any of that.

Just as the balls of mist in the sky would appear, they would also thin out and vanish—a reminder of life on earth. I am simply a mist, here today and gone tomorrow. I've always struggled with obsessing over circumstances in this life, but sometimes, thinking about my own mortality is helpful.

My favorite musical album of all time is Flyleaf's *Memento Mori,* and even the title was always fascinating to me. Remember that you will die. Remember that this life is temporary.

As I lay there that day, I remember thinking that although I don't have to fear death—thanks be to Jesus—I still want to be a good steward of the time I've been given, not out of obligation but out of love, reverence, and gratitude.

Of course, I'm human. I'll always find things to complain about. I used to think it was disrespectful to complain or be brutally honest with God. Turns out, as displayed in many of the Psalms, God not only tolerates that kind of honesty but *welcomes* it.

It's only natural that I would spend a good amount of my life questioning why I have an unusual speech impediment and why God won't heal it, despite countless prayers over many years. The same goes for why He hasn't healed my eyes from always burning or why He doesn't just snap His fingers and make my anxiety and every other struggle go away. That would make things easy and ideal, but I've come to believe these things are meant to be the metaphorical thorn in my side to help keep me humble. That's my headcanon. God's power shines brighter when He uses someone like me in all my weaknesses in order to accomplish His will.

> So to keep me from becoming proud, I was given a thorn in my flesh, a messenger from Satan to torment me and keep me from becoming proud. Three different times I begged the Lord to take it away. Each time he said, "My grace is all you need. My power works best in weakness." So now I am glad to boast about my weaknesses, so that the power of Christ can work through me. That's why I take pleasure in my weaknesses, and in the insults, hardships, persecutions, and troubles that I suffer for Christ. For when I am weak, then I am strong (2 Cor. 12:7-10).

It's not about me or vain, foolish pride. If my speech impediment suddenly went away, I can easily see myself falling into that trap, especially since I already struggle with selfishness as it is. Even though it makes life a lot harder than it needs to be and gives people unlimited ammo to mock me, none of that matters in the end. I'm here today and gone tomorrow. I'd rather have an impaired tongue and humble heart than be physically eloquent and haughty.

I said in an earlier chapter that I've mostly accepted my predicament in the area of speech. *Mostly* was the key word. It's still a daily struggle. It's still incredibly scary to speak on camera, appear on podcasts, or even talk on the phone with people who aren't used to the way I sound. It took the majority of my life to even get close to a place of acceptance, but God is working in me. If He wants to use me to speak, He is more than able. Moses also had a speech impediment, and God used him to be the voice for his people. Even with Aaron's help, I imagine using someone like Moses pointed to God's glory more powerfully than an already well-spoken person would have. The Lord of the universe is infinitely bigger than my insecurities and crippled tongue.

This was a wonderful season, without a doubt. That first handful of years being a Christian was nothing short of miraculous. But things would soon start to collapse, and I would no longer be that enthusiastic, hands-in-the-air type at church. I wouldn't be an always-happy, always-putting-myself-out-there butterfly anymore, despite everything God had done. Is that even allowed? For too long, I believed it wasn't.

# PART THREE
*An Autistic Walk With God*

# CHAPTER FOURTEEN
## How Could I Let This Happen Again?

"Hey, do you wanna join us in prayer?" a friendly girl asked. "We're just praying about random stuff!"

"Oh? Me? Sure!"

I sat down in their little circle on the dorm lobby's floor after Bible study as we prayed about whatever was on our hearts. She had short hair with green bangs, the warmest demeanor, and a highly contagious laugh. I wouldn't have guessed that this specific moment of being invited to a brief prayer circle would lead to a beautiful, lasting friendship with that girl.

Taylor was always a ray of sunshine who helped everyone feel included and brought fun and laughter into every situation. We met sophomore year at InterVarsity and really bonded at one of their conferences. She followed me to Chi Alpha later on. We became roommates, and she was eventually the maid of honor at my wedding. Not to mention, she was my loyal screamo karaoke buddy.

After I graduated from college, she was one of the very few friends who stayed in town for another year. We'd have Friday night "Jesus dates" with our fun coloring Bibles and worship music, praying with and for each other. Those nights were crucial. It was a crazy season of life, where I was working multiple jobs every day of the week, trying to make sure it was safe before attempting to break free from The Dictator and other toxic people, dealing with all new levels of anxiety and the resulting stomach issues, planning my wedding, working out constantly for said wedding because society required me to be skinnier than I was, remaining active in Chi Alpha and trying to see friends as frequently as possible, and also remembering to sleep and maybe occasionally breathe. Most of it didn't bother me, though. Messy and painful stuff aside, life was still exciting and eventful. And for a time, I felt like I was absolutely killing it spiritually.

But then Taylor moved away. Other friends moved away. Following my wedding, hardly anyone I knew remained.

That's a hard thing about living in a transient college town. It's rare that people stick around after finishing school. I was one of the very few who did, and it started getting lonely fast.

Despite my love for Chi Alpha and Akechi's internship with them, I reached a point where I felt too old and out of place for a student ministry. Hardly anyone from my time there was left, and I was in a different stage of life. Regretfully, I decided it was finally time to go.

It turned out it wasn't just an age thing. I found myself just not wanting to socialize at all or do anything that involved getting off the couch. I felt the most comfortable at home and never wanted to leave. Even going to my local church felt like a chore. Big gatherings were exhausting, and I could only survive by mentally teleporting somewhere else.

Before I knew it, I found that the extrovert in me had died. I certainly wasn't back to the way I was pre-Christ, but I found myself—for lack of a better word—relapsing into certain old habits and preferences. In time, it became evident that it was much more than a loss of extroversion.

Though I swore it would never happen again, I fell into a deep depression. But unlike my former sad and angry self, it was apathy this time. After all the madness of life settled down, I figured I just got whiplash. Life became painfully mundane and boring. My exciting schedule turned into a single item on repeat: go to work.

Life stopped, and I stopped with it. I desperately missed the variety I had in college. There was so much more than just my day job and always something to look forward to—usually a church event later in the day or the week or a plan to get together with a group of people for some kind of adventure. I could always hang out with friends at a moment's notice. There was more to life than sitting in an office for forty hours a week, talking to strangers all day, going home exhausted and brain-dead, going to bed, then rinse and repeat. It's hard to explain the contradiction of being bored and overwhelmed at the same time, but that was the cave I lived in.

I was happily married and immensely thankful for that, but I couldn't go on denying that life was losing its flavor in every other way. That was the first domino.

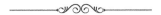

My days turned into the following: it's dark and early. My hair isn't brushed. My eyes are still adorned with morning crust. I'm wearing a hoodie with paint stains, baggy sweatpants, and cheap sneakers that are visibly falling apart. This was not my usual look for work—until it became my usual look for work. I enter the office, manage to utter a grunt of acknowledgment to coworkers, and have just enough mental strength to stare blankly at my computer while contemplating what I'm even doing anymore, desperately craving rest that I wasn't allowed to have and wasn't supposed to need.

This wasn't the plan. I was supposed to be an ultra-professional who had it all together, able to handle anything. But the dominos kept falling, taking my level of caring down with them.

I started gaining weight like crazy, mainly because I was sick to death of dieting constantly for twelve years and couldn't take it anymore. I never wanted to see another vegetable again. In due time, I was back to being the "pumpkin face" of my youth, heavier than ever before, easily able to imagine what certain people would say if they saw me. I couldn't wear makeup anymore due to increasing sensory issues, particularly in my highly sensitive eyes. My eyebrows were becoming patchier by the day due to my struggles with trichotillomania (compulsive hair pulling). Given my history, being required to leave my safe place five times a week and be looked at with judgment felt like a forty-year sentence to silent, inescapable scrutiny and degradation.

Shallow appearance stuff aside, I couldn't be the vivacious ball of sunshine I once was. Try as I might to keep acting like a peppy *Animal Crossing* villager even when I wasn't feeling it, the stamina wasn't there. It didn't help that my embarrassing obsessions with fictional characters were switching into high gear, breaking out of the basement I'd locked them into. I spent most of my remaining mental energy trying to fight them off, to no avail.

Even just the physical act of going *to* work took everything out of me. Actually doing my job was often out of the question. My ability to participate in social interactions was rapidly declining, and my brain couldn't keep up anymore. I was a chronic zombie and didn't have the understanding, much less the language, to describe what was going on and why I could no longer do things.

*Probably because I'm trash,* I thought. *Probably because I'm lazy and selfish. Probably because I'm a terrible person—the ultimate sinner, far worse and more embarrassing than any other.*

Shame was sinking its venomous claws in, locking me into a cell composed of icy concrete where I tried to hide from people and God. It seemed I belonged in there. I thought I was ugly all over again. I was losing social skills and I could never seem to turn off or pray away my intense daydreaming, even with things like therapy and medication. My stuff was too weird to talk about. No one understood. No Christian loves all this geeky stuff as deeply and passionately as I do.

I found myself falling into the clutches of legalism, but only for myself. Everyone else was saved by Christ alone, but me? I'd better get my act together immediately. Re-entering the struggle with genuine human connections sent me back into the frigid embrace of despair. What kind of Christian am I if I can't love my neighbor correctly? I was no longer one of the people at church being physically expressive and enthusiastic during worship, which I attributed to a lack of joy that I ought to hate myself for.

The only times my brain came alive were when I was engaging in special interests. But they weren't "godly" things, so I was supposed to be resisting temptation and "worldly" pleasures. That was the proper Christian thing to do, as I understood it.

No one disagreed or said anything to the contrary when I was calling myself a filthy idolater because I liked things a lot. So clearly, something was very, very wrong with me. I needed to repent. I needed prayers for deliverance—obviously.

The more I tried to push forward with this mentality, even with prayer and accountability, the more I declined. Apart from things like scorpions and chronic pain, this kind of relapse was probably my biggest fear in life, and I was watching it unfold into reality. I was reverting back to *that* person—the one who was hated, ridiculed, unacceptable, and unworthy of dignity or of taking up space in a world that clearly belongs to the fun, loud, "normal" people.

My husband was always supportive, which I'm forever grateful for. But in that season, I drowned it out with my blaring self-hatred. My happy cheeriness and quick wit had vaporized. My interest in people and activities that were socially acceptable kept decreasing by the day, while I couldn't stop loving my interests that were not socially acceptable, no matter how embarrassing it felt, even after prayerfully and aggressively pushing them away and thinking I had "victory" over them. I needed to hide from both God and His people, unable to show my face until I repented and overcame everything that made me a weird sinner.

*How could I allow all of this to happen again? What's wrong with me? I should know better! All I have to do is stop doing and thinking about all the things I enjoy forever. Why can't I manage that simple task?*

I was driving home from a Bible study one night, where I had been continually feeling ignored, excluded, and overall out of place but was trying to smile and push through it, anyway. And then I couldn't anymore. I unwillingly broke down bawling in the car.

"It's happening again! Please, God, I don't want to feel alone again. Don't let me be an outcast again. I don't *ever* want to go back to that place!"

For so many years, I truly believed that God had completely taken my autism away. After all, I had experienced a lot of sudden, dramatic changes. I had a very limited, often very false understanding of what autism even is. But in these difficult, confusing years, I started to wonder if perhaps He took aspects of it away, if that's even a thing. But maybe I was still on the spectrum. Maybe I was painfully mistaken all that time.

This was eventually confirmed when I sought a professional and received my diagnosis. After four years of crashing and burning at a wide variety of jobs, I'd come to my wit's end. I needed to know what was happening to my brain. The diagnosis provided an answer, and I needed to sit with it for a while.

Post-diagnosis, I sought to learn as much as I could about what autism actually is. I discovered what things like masking and ableism are. I learned that I never should've been forced to wear a neurotypical mask and play pretend twenty-four seven. I never should've been unrealistically expected to do things as a disabled person exactly like everyone else, nor should I have been looked down upon whenever I couldn't pull it off.

I was always being forced, whether directly or indirectly, to be "normal," and therefore wanted that more than anything. It was a bit devastating learning that I never would be, no matter how hard I might try. But then came the time to ask why letting my brain operate the way it's wired was such a crime. Memoirs by other autistic authors have been invaluable. Identifying parallels in the stories of others, really driving home the point that it's not just me, has given me a sense of validation I never thought possible.

At long last, I had my answer. I was not only experiencing regular burnout, but *autistic* burnout. All those years of intense masking and forcefully putting myself out there, trying to cram myself into a mold I was never meant to fit into, did a number on me and I had no idea. It truly was as if I had actually lost certain skills, which is what often happens in the autistic burnout phenomenon. Regardless of determination and attitude, there were things I simply could not handle anymore. I finally had to acknowledge the damage to my shape from years of violently trying to jam my square-pegged self into society's round hole. No matter how much I cut away at the sides and corners, I was never going to fit.

When people are diagnosed late after a lifetime of masking, there are usually questions of, "Who am I *really*, then?" I, on the other hand, was far more curious about my former self. I had allowed the imposter to stay, but she fled and remains a mystery.

How did I live out such an outgoing, fearless, loud existence during college? Who was that person? Deep down, was I just trying to prove to the world and to myself that I was capable? Maybe it was influence or the freedom high. Perhaps it was denial due to internalized ableism. I'd assume all of the above. God only knows.

This whole season kept me wondering, *In what universe would I even be allowed to be depressed or be anything but happy and peppy? Seriously, what right do I have? God has blessed me abundantly and saved me from so many things. I'm happily married to my favorite person. I have a roof over my head and never have to worry about where my next meal is coming from. How dare I be anything other than happy!*

I knew there were plenty of biblical figures who experienced depression and sorrow (just look at David in many of the Psalms). But apparently, when it's me, it's not okay. It was as if there was a list of qualifications to be met in order to be allowed to feel how I felt or to struggle in any way. Or there were different levels of suffering to be achieved in life before being granted the key to unlock a chest that contained permission to feel hurt. I guess I've had that mentality ingrained in me pretty much my whole life, now that I think about it.

*Other people have it so much worse than me, so anything and everything I feel is invalid. What right do I have to experience negative thoughts and emotions when things could always be worse? I'm privileged; therefore, I can't ever be unhappy about anything. I'm an ungrateful brat.*

And I actually don't think this is just a me thing. We get a lot of those kinds of messages from culture, dressed up in different styles.

Much of it turned back into a colorful variety of self-loathing, especially pre-diagnosis. I hated that I couldn't go back to the way I used to be, as even my ability to fake it evaporated. No one likes a Negative Nelly—or, as they say these days, "Positive vibes only," right? So surely, I shouldn't be hanging around people until I got myself together.

Believing that lie frequently kept me in hiding whenever it wasn't absolutely necessary to leave home. I saw myself as the ultimate failure of a human being. All those years of growing and bettering myself, all just to come crashing down in the end. Was it all an illusion?

I thought that "shining the light of Christ to the world" meant that I had to always be a personification of the sun. Other people, I was always told, were supposed to see my outward joy and crave God as a result. It was my responsibility. On the flip side, depression wasn't allowed because it was a sign that I wasn't content enough in the Lord. Onlookers supposedly won't want to seek God if they see me struggling and upset because what kind of a sales pitch is that? If people in my life reject Him, it must be my fault for doing something wrong or not putting in enough effort.

It's amazing how gifted my mind is at incorrectly piecing together messages that were never intended. It clings to any reason it can find for me to hide from God, as if He can't see me when I'm under the covers.

Despite all the times He had proven it over and over, this season and my downfall caused me to question the Lord's love for me, His rich grace and mercy, and even whether I could lose my salvation if I didn't get it together again. Of all my anxieties, that one is the absolute worst place to be. The accuser wants me there. He's a liar.

My default is to expect punishment whenever I mess up or struggle—or get a condescending lecture, at the very least. On a good day, it would be something like this: "Ha! I told you so! You got what you deserve! That's right, come crawling back to me now in shame, you disgraceful, pitiful thing. If only you had done what I said and done it perfectly, maybe you wouldn't be in such a sorry state. That's what you get for not being good enough. Now, let me blissfully drink from my wine glass as I gloat and watch in satisfaction as you writhe in agony on the floor."

Or perhaps on a not so good day: "Who do you think you are, coming back now after what you did? How *dare* you. You have no right asking for help. I'm going to make you pay. Get ready to spend the rest of your life making up for your mistakes. Further failure will not be tolerated. Oh? You're in pain? Good!"

Neither of these are God. It's so easy to feel like God is disappointed in us or somehow loves us less when we sin or are in low seasons. Dane Ortlund counters this and goes into depth on the topic in his must-read book *Gentle and Lowly*: "The cumulative testimony of the four Gospels is that when Jesus Christ sees the fallenness of the world all about him, his deepest impulse, his most natural instinct, is to move toward that sin and suffering, not away from it."[3]

Yet despite what Scripture tells me about God's unchanging love for me, I'm always vigorously searching for reasons why I might be unacceptable to Him—just in case. It's always the what ifs.

One of the biggest ways I've fought against all of this has been learning about my autistic brain—which God gave me—and getting to a place of not only acceptance but appreciation for it.

————————oɔ⌇⊙⊙⌇ɔ————————

Let's talk about empathy. I got my degree in social work because I wanted to help people. I wanted to serve. I wanted to love. So why, starting in this season, was I suddenly so nightmarishly bad at empathy and compassion? Why did going out of one's way to help another seem to come so naturally to everyone except for me? Why did I never know what to say or do with information someone gave me about their problems? The only logical answer was that I'm a bad person.

I didn't really stop to consider that maybe it's at least partly related to my burnout and slower processing times. Of course, being in denial for so long about still being autistic didn't help.

While I hate the stereotype that autistic people can't be empathetic (which is absolutely not true, in case you were wondering), I also think it's an overcorrection and another overgeneralization, just in the opposite direction, to say that *all* autistic people actually feel empathy *too* strongly. We're all different. It's still a reality that some people can have a harder time with it. At the very least, many of us struggle with showing it and responding in expected ways.

As a Christian, it often makes me feel disgusting inside, knowing that I'm called to love all people all the time in every situation—as if loving people always has to be an outward show. I wanted to bury myself in the sand whenever I saw a non-Christian display seemingly better kindness and empathy for others than I did or when my clients were visibly nicer to people than I, the one who was supposed to be a professional in the realm of compassion, ever thought to be. I would then beat myself down for being more concerned about my lack of feelings and failure to take action than I was about the person in question. It was the most ironic kind of vicious cycle. I concluded that I was a failure as a Christian and as a person—a poser who's unqualified to talk about Christ or be His follower. You gotta love the work of the accuser. (I'm actually not a fan of his work at all.)

But here's the thing: a non-empathetic person wouldn't care about being bad at empathy. Struggling with it differs greatly from it being nonexistent or impossible, like the stereotype often implies. The fact that I have a heart always wanting to grow and love people better is, I believe, one piece of evidence that I *am* an empathetic person. But even more so, empathy can look different from person to person. Much like autism itself, empathy is not a cookie-cutter, one-size-fits-all thing. Just because someone doesn't outwardly show it doesn't necessarily mean it's not there.

When I think about it, why is empathy always expected to be a performance? For all you know, maybe I'm weeping for you in my mind and praying for you without actually saying it or showing emotion. Or maybe I'm not thinking or feeling much right there in the moment, but I will later that day or that week. Maybe I'll feel it deeply once it sinks in after some time. I may not always fall apart at sad stories and be full of encouraging things to say, and I may not immediately recognize when someone needs help and instinctively drop everything to lend a hand, as most people probably would. But that doesn't mean I'm not empathetic.

As much as I love gaming, the comparison game is a dangerous one that I wouldn't recommend to anyone—zero out of ten stars. This can sometimes include comparing yourself to yourself. After being saved, I was basically always cheerful for almost a decade straight. It was awesome. Even when hard and painful circumstances arose, I never lost heart. I always held onto God and looked for the positive in every situation. Optimism was my default. So why couldn't I do that anymore? I should know better, right? What happened?

Besides burnout, honestly, I don't really know. Perhaps it was spiritual warfare or past traumas catching up with me. It's probably a number of things. "You should know better" has become one of my least favorite sayings on the planet, at least in these types of contexts. It's not always that simple.

But one thing I know now is there's nothing shameful about being autistic, an introvert, or being more on the quiet side. It doesn't decrease a person's worth. There is actually great value in those things. My past and the lies I was told don't change that fact. Often, the quietest people have the loudest minds and the coolest ideas.

Susan Cain goes into depth about the value of quiet people and introverts in her hugely successful book *Quiet: The Power of Introverts in a World That Can't Stop Talking*. One quote that sticks out in my mind is this:

> If you're an introvert, you also know that the bias against quiet can cause deep psychic pain. As a child you might have overheard your parents apologize for your shyness. ("Why can't you be more like the Kennedy boys?" the Camelot-besotted parents of one man I interviewed repeatedly asked him.) Or at school you might have been prodded to come "out of your shell"—that noxious expression which fails to appreciate that some animals naturally carry shelter everywhere they go, and that some humans are just the same.[4]

Being loud and extroverted is not the only valid way to live, despite what society likes to say or imply. Our culture wants every person to be an outgoing ball of energy who's always the life of the party, but imagine if that actually happened: the absolute, never-ending chaos. Not everyone can be the life of the party, or there would be no such thing. People aren't all supposed to be the same. Some of us were Divinely created to have those personalities, and others of us were Divinely created to be soft-spoken and laid back, or anywhere in between. One way of being is not inherently superior.

--------‐◦∕◦⊙◦⌒◦--------

With how deeply the toxic productivity mentality is baked into my bones, you'd think my childhood home would've had a sign with this inspirational message hanging in the kitchen: "Get over it. No wimps allowed in this house. Life is pain, and you just need to deal. No resting because that's lazy. Make yourself useful at all times, no matter what. If you think you've done enough, you haven't. Earn your right to exist."

Even if that wasn't completely unreasonable on its own, sometimes I just get to a place where I'm spent—not just my body but my brain. I can only keep up the tough act for so long. Sometimes I need to take time off to rest and recharge—more than what the average person requires. I don't have the same energy levels, sensory tolerance, or mental stamina as other people. We're all different, and I'm learning that it's actually okay.

I think a lot of us neurodivergent folk feel we need to have the mindset of, "I don't let my disability stop me!" It's been drilled in. But the reality is that for many of us, there will be moments, days, and seasons where it *does* stop us. And we shouldn't have to feel bad about it or agree with ableist views and agendas. We wouldn't get mad at someone with a broken or amputated ankle for not being able to run track like the rest of the students in gym class. We wouldn't label them as lazy. Considering how demanding and stimulating the world is, we neurodivergents often need extra rest and different kinds of rest than our neurotypical peers. We should allow ourselves that. We are not defined by our productivity. It's okay to not always be great at everything that life demands. This applies to anyone, disabled or not.

Though it took a very long time, I've also learned that it's okay to cut toxic people out of our lives when we need to. Yes, even for Christians who are supposed to love people. Love does not equate to enabling harmful behavior. I've had to learn that the hard way many times. I've been demonized for leaving abusive situations and refusing to return. It's unfortunate, but I've had to remind myself time and time again that my safety and mental health are more important than those people's opinions. "Don't befriend angry people or associate with hot-tempered people, or you will learn to be like them and endanger your soul" (Prov. 22:24-25).

Regardless of what we struggle with, God loves us no less. He loves me just as much when I'm lying on the couch playing on my phone or wallowing in sadness as He does when I'm worshiping at church. He sees us in our struggles. He is with us in them, even when we feel alone. We never need to hide. In His grace, He invites us to come to Him as we are.

None of us will ever be perfect on this side of Heaven, no matter how "Christian" we become. We shouldn't put that expectation on ourselves. Our behaviors aren't what save us. Even when I do find myself backsliding into unhealthy habits and thought patterns, I'm still a renewed and ransomed child of God. That will never change. "However, those the Father has given me will come to me, and I will *never* reject them" (John 6:37, emphasis mine).

Happiness and all other emotions are always changing with circumstances, but joy in the Lord is constant, whether it's outwardly visible or not. Even when I'm down and stuck, I'm alive in Christ.

# CHAPTER FIFTEEN
## When It's Less Easy

My breathing is heavy. I feel a knot in my throat and a ticking bomb in my stomach. I can picture the color leaving my face as I try to stop the racing thoughts that are rapidly spiraling out of control. My chest tightens as the weight of a boulder presses down, while loud whispers in my mind viciously taunt my weakened state, now wide open to attacks.

*This is the end. You really messed up this time. And that other time. And that other time. You are repulsive and unforgivable. You'll spend the rest of your life paying for being who you are and for making this mistake. And the next one. Even if it wasn't your fault, it's always your fault. Even if you didn't mean to hurt anyone, of course you did, you insensitive imbecile. This is who you really are. If only people knew the "real" you, not a single soul would ever love you.*

These assaults on my mind are common when shame, fear, and trauma get together and go bowling. They are all professional superstars at the sport, and I am the pins. The whole thing becomes a hyperfixation—a convenient foothold for the accuser, I'd say. This is an example of an area where hyperfixation can be a bad thing—not just weird or annoying to onlookers, but actually harmful.

Though I'm not exactly thrilled to admit it, to this day, I still struggle severely with confrontation in any form. Even the slightest hint of a negative interaction, criticism, or change in tone can send me into a panic. I immediately feel small and defenseless, always defaulting to flight over fight and assuming the worst possible outcome. I was conditioned to be spineless and always do as I'm told, no matter what. No arguing allowed. No differing opinions allowed. It's disrespectful, and punishment awaits.

In the midst of hostile conversation, even when there's no yelling, my mind tends to freeze up completely due to overwhelm, and I can't process—a form of autistic shutdown. But these things are unavoidable in life. Even when I try to always be chill and agreeable, kind at all times, and never one to argue, it's still inevitable to some extent.

When I became a Christian, I was oblivious to the reality that I would be despised by many for it. I'm thankful that God shielded me from that during my early years, as I was a lot more fragile then. Since I was already disliked and isolated in my non-Christian days, I'm not sure if I'd be able to handle any more of that so soon.

I wasn't expecting to eventually lose dear friends and get kicked out of their lives for being a Christian, whether or not I ever talked about it, or to be actively harassed in professional settings for being a church-goer instead of a wild party animal. Ultimately, I didn't know that I was expected to shut up about my "religion" and keep my joy to myself. But these kinds of things, as infuriating and heartbreaking as they are in the moment, have actually led to a lot of growth in the long run. And for that reason, I'm grateful.

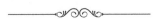

"Keep your religion to yourself!"

I mean, to be fair, I kind of get it. If I wasn't a Christian, I'd probably be saying the same thing. Ever since I came to know God, it has crushed my heart to know that there are people who don't know His love and who are actively against Him. Their reasons why are often understandable, which is even more saddening. I've always been aware of this reality; but sometimes, it really sinks in and breaks me—especially when it's people I know and love personally. My heart's desire is for everyone to know Christ's great love and experience joy like I have and that people would want to know Him without feeling forced or obligated. The key word there is *without*. I believe that love honors freedom.

While I never want to be forceful or obnoxious, keeping it to myself in every way doesn't make a ton of sense to me, the more I think about it. It's the most central part of who I am, and my identity in Christ is exactly that: an *identity*, not just a label. Similar to autism, my faith is a core part of my entire being and is going to at least occasionally come out naturally when I talk, regardless of who I'm talking to. Even just fun, personal anecdotes are often directly connected to God or church somehow. Asking someone to keep it to themselves and pretend it doesn't exist is, in my view, not much different from asking them to suppress any other part of their identity as a person. (Please don't ask me or anyone else to suppress our neurodivergence around you. We'd appreciate that.)

I've often heard faith being talked about as if it's just some side thing that Christians do for fun—as if it's something we're supposed to keep confidential, like a secret part-time job where we go in once a week and then hide all the evidence when we get home. But God is everything. He is with us wherever we go and is involved in every aspect of our lives.

It's not about religion and formalities. My faith started off with a relationship with God before I even knew the rules, and that's what's kept it alive. People have different opinions on this, but I'm personally not fond of the word "religion" when referring to God because it usually makes people think of a bunch of strict rules and legalism. That's not the point. We wouldn't be devout lovers of our spouses, children, friends, or anyone else if the relationship was only based on a set of rules, would we? I mean . . . I certainly wouldn't. Rules and boundaries are important and helpful, but those aren't the main focus of genuine, loving bonds.

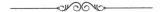

I know it's hard when we don't understand everything God does or doesn't do. I have a lot of empathy for people with earnest questions and concerns. I myself often have a bunch of question marks floating above my head when I read through Scripture, like a whole comic book character. Especially the Old Testament, with all the wrath and violence. My autistic brain also tends to struggle greatly with poetry and anything that's deeply metaphorical rather than straightforward. I ask questions and try to look deeper into it, but I won't lie—I still hurt myself in confusion, and I don't like not having all the answers.

But despite that, I like to think about it like a young child who has legitimately (read: *legitimately*) good, loving parents, and the kid doesn't always understand everything Mom and Dad do or say. Maybe some things feel unfair. Maybe it seems to contradict their loving nature when they get angry and discipline the child. Do anger and discipline make those parents heartless monsters? Or does that idea contradict what the child already knows to be true of them? Because of their healthy relationship that already exists, the child can ultimately trust that their parents are still good, having only their best interests in mind, despite not understanding everything. Just because this kid doesn't know every last thing about their parents and their character doesn't mean they're not loving and trustworthy. Whether we like it or not, we're still small kids in the grand scheme of things, no matter how much wisdom and intellect we acquire.

When my parent dropped me off on that first day of preschool and I lost my mind and threw literal hours of tantrums, I wondered how someone who supposedly loved me could possibly abandon me there. I couldn't conceive of the idea that it was for my own good—the beginning of getting an education. Any explanations my toddler self was given didn't make sense. All I saw was that I was abandoned. But sure enough, my parent came back. Like those stressful and overwhelming school days, I'm here now with all my questions and fears, waiting for my Father to come pick me up and take me home. (The stuff that happened later with my family is beside the point. God doesn't change.)

It doesn't contradict a loving parent's nature to do things out of genuine love that we don't always like or understand. So it is with God. I'm called to trust Him even when I can't possibly wrap my head around things. I've always hated uncertainty and not having all the answers or being told, "I'll tell you when you're older" (or when we get to Heaven, in this case). But that's often how it is. I frequently need to put down my pride and impatient attitude of demanding answers immediately. As Proverbs 3:5-6 advises, "Trust in the Lord with all your heart; do not depend on your own understanding. Seek his will in all you do, and he will show you which path to take."

God saved me both in this life and in the life to come and continually amazes me throughout the years with His goodness and glory. This is why I'm so passionate. My faith isn't just some obligation or something I was brainwashed into. It wasn't me picking up a Bible one day and randomly deciding to base my life on it. And it wasn't from going to church, as I always zoned out when I was forced to go and couldn't tell you a single thing I remember being preached back then. (Remember how shaken I was when I heard the word "sin" for the first time . . . as a junior in high school?) I was basically on my own for a while after becoming a Christian. No one was telling me to pursue God, yet I wanted Him more than anything. He is my ultimate Identity.

"But, Miya," I hear you say, "religion is a choice! You're not born that way, so it can't be an identity like other things can."

My answer to this type of comment is yes and no. Yes, it's a choice to pursue God, both initially and in our everyday lives. Love is an ongoing choice, after all. You don't come out of the womb automatically a willing Christ-follower. However, we're told in Scripture that once we receive Christ, He becomes our Identity. We see this in the following passages:

- "This means that anyone who belongs to Christ has become a new person. The old life is gone; a new life has begun" (2 Cor. 5:17).
- "My old self has been crucified with Christ. It is no longer I who live, but Christ lives in me. So I live in this earthly body by trusting in the Son of God, who loved me and gave himself for me" (Gal. 2:20).
- "But to all who believed him and accepted him, he gave the right to become children of God" (John 1:12).

On top of that, I would argue that after God's intervention in my heart, I could never, in my right mind, go back to the way I was before. He has saturated me from the inside out. Mere labels alone don't do that.

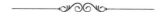

My ability to not take things personally is like my motorcycle. I don't have a motorcycle. As someone who's always been canceled and ghosted for reasons never explained, I don't always love living in an era of cancel culture's extreme popularity. In a time where everything is offensive, it's hard to not be afraid of saying . . . anything, really. Maybe my struggles with unspoken cues and impulsive bluntness have something to do with it, but I could say something completely random and innocent and come to find out later that it was actually deeply offensive to some. Sometimes, it legitimately was, in which case I completely take it back, repent of my ignorance, and try to do better next time. Other times, I'm shamed for not overcomplicating a simple comment and not imagining every possible scenario where it might offend someone somewhere in the world before I spoke or for not thinking about the small chance that someone might misinterpret the comment and twist it to make it mean something else entirely.

Now people are furious with me, and the panic and guilt stay in me for several days (or years). I often make myself sick from it. It encourages me to revert to my old ways: just hide and stay quiet all the time. Don't say a word. It's the safest option.

Though, I guess as an autistic person, I probably *do* say some blunt, off-putting things sometimes and am oblivious. Sometimes, weird stuff I don't even mean flies out of my mouth, and I wonder why on earth I said it. That's something I'm always trying to work on, but it doesn't help when no one tells me I upset them and I'm simply expected to win the guessing game.

The thing is, being hated by people is inevitable in life. Nothing and no one is universally liked. Even the sweetest, most caring people will upset somebody at some point. Jesus Himself was offensive because He boldly proclaimed truth, not worried about some people getting offended by it (looking at you, Pharisees). He even tells us straight up that we'll be hated by the world if we follow Him: "'If the world hates you, remember that it hated me first. The world would love you as one of its own if you belonged to it, but you are no longer part of the world. I chose you to come out of the world, so it hates you'" (John 15:18-19).

Of course, this does *not* mean that we can just say whatever horrible things we want to people, "in the name of Jesus." That's a hard no. We cannot abuse Scripture and use it as an excuse to bully, shame, and dehumanize others. *That* is taking the Lord's name in vain. I wish I could personally apologize to every person who has ever had these verses and concepts used against them in hateful, traumatizing ways. Christian, if this is you, check your heart and repent.

Even though I am, in all honesty, spineless most of the time when it comes to confrontation and my anxiety goes through the roof and into space, I will stand firm in Christ. On a good day, my backbone has the strength of a Pocky stick, but I still won't deny the Lord of my life.

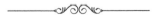

Many of you are probably already thinking this, so I'll get to it. I know that in this day and age, no one wants to hear a Christian in America whine about experiencing hardships—something about it being a first-world problem. In all fairness, yeah—worse things absolutely happen in life. It can be good to remind ourselves of that for the purposes of appreciating what we have and widening our perspectives. It can also inspire us to take action and help others in whatever ways we're able. But when the reminder becomes shame-based or weaponized, it goes back to the idea that anyone who lives in fortunate circumstances to any degree has no right to ever be upset about anything because it could always be worse.

There are people who share my experiences with cultural opposition to faith, but it's not universal by any means. In some areas, it's just the opposite. In other areas, it's unimaginably worse. But ultimately, the fact that worse things happen doesn't erase the reality that painful stuff takes place in the lives of Christ-followers in various areas and on different levels, even if it seems minimal to some. We all have our own lives and our own problems as human beings in a broken world. It's always painful to lose precious people in our lives, regardless of the reason why. On one hand, being mistreated or canceled is not the same as literal persecution, and it would be completely absurd to claim otherwise. But on the other, it doesn't need to become a suffering competition. No one needs to obtain the key to a locked chest, granting permission to be sad. It's so easy to feel guilty when comparing our pain to that of other people, but that doesn't mean it's invalid.

I still wrestle with this regularly. There will always be somebody somewhere who has it worse, but that doesn't mean we aren't allowed to feel our pain or talk about it. By that logic, no one would ever have permission. Sometimes, I feel like I need to post this on my mirror: "If someone gets mad at me because they don't think whatever pain I'm expressing is brutal enough to count, that's their problem. Let them be mad. Move on."

Saying things can be dangerous. Historically, I'd default to being quiet to be on the safe side, but I've noticed that some people will likewise promote the idea that silence is violence. Don't speak up, but don't *not* speak up. Don't have any opinions or beliefs because you're wrong, but get out there and make your voice heard, or you're part of the problem. I don't know how to solve this Rubik's Cube. Send help.

We can't control how others see us, regardless of what we do or don't do. And that's okay. We can only control our own actions and attitudes and remember our own worth.

While I was writing this book, I frequently showed parts of it to Akechi and asked, "Does this sound offensive? Will people hate my guts for saying this?" I know full well that no matter what I could possibly say, it's going to offend somebody somewhere. People could even take this sentence right here and twist it to mean something different if they want to. It's all out of my control. So I'm trying (with varying levels of success) not to worry about that so much and just focusing on being honest with where I've been and where I'm at.

All of this is to say, if I'm going to be hated, I would far rather it be for my faith—the God who saved my life—than anything else. I'm supposed to consider it great joy, after all. "'God blesses you when people mock you and persecute you and lie about you and say all sorts of evil things against you because you are my followers. Be happy about it! Be very glad! For a great reward awaits you in heaven. And remember, the ancient prophets were persecuted in the same way'" (Matt. 5:11-12).

I've experienced so much inexplicable joy in my heart that never would've been if it weren't for the Lord. He makes life worth it every day that I wake up—even on the heavier days when I don't really want to wake up. Yes, there will be times of suffering, and things won't always be easy. There will always be opposition to my faith in some way or another, whether it's in the form of harassment, exclusion, spiritual attacks, or whatever else. But it's worth it. If nothing else, we're promised in several places in Scripture that we'll be rewarded if we persevere to the end.

One of the countless things God has taught me is to be thankful and not lose sight of what I have. I know I've done the cliché thing of using nature as illustrations a few times, but I've always been one who prefers to stay inside most of the time. I feel the safest and most content when I'm indoors. We don't have to go out into a forest or hike a tall mountain in order to see God's glory. It's everywhere. Even when I'm just lying on the couch and looking at the walls that surround me, I'm filled with so much gratitude. God has given me shelter. I'm so thankful to have a place to live where I'm safe and healthy. I'm a mere sinful blob of dust, and God doesn't owe me anything. Yet He takes care of me abundantly. If it weren't for the Lord of my heart, I would take all that I have for granted and feel entitled to always have more. Nothing would've ever been enough.

I sometimes feel regretful for not pursuing God for the first almost fifteen years of my life. But all the same, I'm so grateful for the journey. I'm glad that I could come to my own decision to follow Jesus. I've gained God-given wisdom because of it and am able to relate to other people who have gone through similar situations, when it all would have otherwise sounded foreign to me.

I would've probably been livid in the midst of the suffering back in my B.C. days, had someone told me it would all be worth it someday. I would write it off as a stupid, overused platitude and that they didn't know what they were talking about because they had never been through what I go through every day. I might've even physically assaulted them and cussed them out if I was that bold and not terrified of the consequences. Cheesy as it may sound, I truly believe I'm an example of how Jesus really can change hearts. Choosing to follow Him was like discovering my true self for the first time. It doesn't matter who we are. He can make masterpieces out of our messes.

# CHAPTER SIXTEEN
## Autistic Traits and Christianity

I feel that I'm at a place where my autism affects me enough to make certain things harder than they are for most people but doesn't *visibly* affect me enough to be considered a disability. There's very little grace from the world when I struggle. It's seen as an excuse, and I'm still expected to perform exactly the same as a neurotypical person at every moment.

But despite the stigma, when you really think about it, is being autistic really so bad? Is it something that even needs "healing" in the first place? The answer is usually a resounding *no* from neurodivergent people, though I've found that it can vary depending on who you talk to, even within the autism community. And it's very true that autism can look and be experienced differently from one person to the next. Some autistic people are completely happy and unashamed of their brains. Others wish to be healed, at least from certain struggles or characteristics. My take is that people are completely allowed to feel how they feel about their own selves, as long as there's no shaming toward others. I've been on both sides, and it took me around twenty-six years to realize the positive and change my mindset.

It all started during a conversation with a wonderful friend and fellow autistic, where I was making ignorant comments and finally being called out on them.

"Yeah, I was autistic at one point, too, but then God healed me!"

"Well . . . Those kinds of comments are what offend people. Most autistic people don't see it as something that needs healing."

"Huh?"

Thus began the journey.

As stated at the beginning, I'm no expert on the matter by any means, but I've come to find that being neurodivergent means that we think differently than other people do. We learn, process, and communicate differently. We have different support needs. It doesn't make us stupid or take away any of our value as humans created in the image of God. Often, the loveliest things about us are a result of our autism. Take away the autism and we'd be different people entirely. It affects everything about us—how we think, feel, react, process information, and perceive the world. It's not just some side thing or a simple personality quirk. It's who we are.

I had many misconceptions in the past, but I no longer believe that autism is something that needs to be healed or cured. I think that idea only causes harm. It promotes the notion that we should be hated and shouldn't exist, and we probably wouldn't if there was a way to intervene (in other words, eugenics). If a magical cure were to hypothetically come about, we would lose ourselves. Someone would have to literally open up our heads, remove our brains, and put someone else's in.

But Jim Sinclair says it much better: "This is what we know, when you tell us of your fondest hopes and dreams for us: that your greatest wish is that one day we will cease to be, and strangers you can love will move in behind our faces."[5]

This is also what many of us hear when Christians say things like, "You can overcome your autism through Christ!" (Please don't say that.)

Some may scratch their heads at the idea of me not wanting to be cured from the disability that brings so much struggle to my life. A lot could be said here, but it's important to note that there's a difference between desiring to be better at a specific skill versus wanting my autism to vanish—at the expense of myself. I'd obviously love to be a stellar conversationalist who can always read the room and not get so easily overwhelmed by the world, but that's not where God has me. Even if I somehow became a master wizard of dialogue and quick wit, that wouldn't mean my autism is suddenly gone. It would be more like the soundboard being adjusted. Most people have *something* they want to struggle with less or a skill they wish to obtain, regardless of their neurology. That's just life. No one is proficient at everything. But why is the focus so often only on the negatives when it comes to neurodivergence?

Sure, a neurotypical person might be better at socializing. But likewise, there are probably other things that a neurodivergent person is better at. For instance, I've noticed throughout my life that writing comes a lot more naturally to me than it does for a lot of my peers, as it's my strongest, preferred method of communication. Hyper-focusing is the reason I was able to not only follow through in completing this book but did so in just a few months (billions of editing rounds aside). As a kid, I typically caught onto computers and technology faster than most of my peers—not to encourage the stereotype, but it happened for me. I can focus extremely well on things that interest me. I'm flowing with creative energy on a regular basis. I'm honest and loyal. I'm able to have different and unique insights into things compared to the loudest and most social people in the group. We all have strengths and weaknesses.

Of course, this isn't to say that our value is dependent on being skilled at something. But it's a gift that we can all see the world in different ways. Different isn't bad. God loves the brains He gave us.

The same goes for "maladaptive" daydreaming—my specialty. Is it really such a bad thing? Or what about intense special interests in general? It's true that these things might cause problems in excess, and it's important to have enough self-control to pull away when we need to focus on something else in the moment or attend to other responsibilities. Special interests and hobbies should be things that richly complement our lives, not completely overtake them. They should help us blossom without utterly consuming us. But ultimately, why is this stuff so looked down upon? What's wrong with enjoying things and being creative?

For so many years, I believed that using my imagination and having special interests were these filthy, disgusting sins I needed to get rid of. I tried *so* hard for years but never succeeded. The couple of times I found short-lived "freedom," it always came back more intensely than before. Innocent, nerdy daydreaming (or mental story writing) seemed like an unshakeable sin. It was happening in my mind, so I couldn't exactly have someone chain me to a chair to prevent me from committing a certain action. Why couldn't I have just been put into suspended animation after I got saved until Christ's return? At least, that way, I wouldn't sin.

I believe all this shame came from church culture, not God Himself. I fell into deep despair for a long time, since I evidently couldn't repent from daydreaming, no matter how spiritually invested I was. But what I was eventually encouraged to question after many agonizing years is unless we're thinking about clearly sinful things and will be tempted to act on them (adultery, murder, thievery, etc.) and as long as we're not neglecting real life responsibilities, then what's the problem? What's wrong with using the creative brains that God gave us?

He is the ultimate Creator, and we're made in His image. Therefore, we reflect His image when we're creative. We wouldn't have movies, books, music, or really any kind of art if it weren't for people's imaginations. When you watch or read a piece of fiction, you're watching or reading someone's daydream. But it's not often that folks label those creators as lazy, useless, terrible people for their creative minds. It's usually just us common folk. If we haven't become famous for it, we're just wasting time in La La Land.

I am still working through this and trying to figure it out. I don't have all the answers. I could be totally off, for all I know. Please keep this in mind as you go and don't take what I say as gospel. These are my convictions and perspectives, but they aren't universal. It's important to follow one's own convictions.

I don't think we always need to label something as bad just because society thinks it's weird or unusual. Church culture in general can have some inconsistent standards sometimes, at least from what I've seen. It's perfectly acceptable to watch sports all day and get all excited and riled up over them, but watching anime or reading fanfiction for that same amount of time is labeled as pointless, idolatry, and laziness. Why is one morally neutral hobby okay but not another?

I know this is controversial, but the reality is that traditional methods alone of connecting with God might not work as well for us neurodivergents as they do for most neurotypicals. That's not to say we shouldn't do them, but maybe there are other activities that help us feel closer to Him as well. I commonly feel close to God when I take time to be still and reflect on all He's done for me—often while listening to music, looking through old photos, or even gaming, as opposed to, say, trying to sit down and shame-read a bunch of theology for hours or getting up early and trying to have scheduled "quiet time" when I'm a zombie and my brain can't focus. Having realistic goals is the only way I've maintained the habit of Bible reading at all. Even listening to worship songs or faith podcasts while doing other things can be effective. One of my favorite things is having discussions with my online faith community.

The traditional, intentional things are extremely important, without a doubt. But we can also talk to God while doing various other activities. Quiet time and theology books are wonderful things, and this is not by any means to say we should neglect reading the Bible or anything like that. I want to be clear that nothing can replace Scripture. It's just that there are so many ways to hang out with Jesus. I don't think it always has to be the same two or three things. I've been lovingly taught that it's not always about the amount of time I spend on one thing versus another. Spending five hours watching a show does not mean that a six-hour Bible reading session is required to make up for it. I spend far more time working, writing, and enjoying my special interests of the moment than going on dates with my husband, but that doesn't mean he's less important to me than those things.

As my mentor once told me, "We don't all have to live like nuns." We don't have to feel like we're not allowed to do anything ever outside of going to church, reading the Bible, telling people about Jesus, and other Christian-y deeds. We often get this message from Church culture that spending time with God is limited to those things, as if He's confined to them. But in reality, He is present with us everywhere in all we do. He doesn't say, "Oh, you're finished reading the Bible for the day? Okay, bye. I'm going away now. Call me back when it's time for your next reading session." He's just as present with me when I'm watching *One Piece* as He is when I'm reading Genesis. He doesn't love us more or less based on the particular activity we're partaking in at that moment. I love my feline children both when they're purring in my lap and when they're off doing their own thing.

Instead of thinking of it from a shame-based perspective, perhaps it would be more helpful for us to remember that any loving relationship is a two-way street. God loves to be with us when we're doing the things we enjoy and experiencing His goodness; but likewise, it would be a loving response on our end to also spend time doing things He likes doing together, and getting to know Him better. It's helpful to find one's own rhythm.

I personally think it's valuable to find the things that work best for us individually and learn how to be intentional with including God in our hobbies and special interests. For instance, I try to maintain the habit of frequently looking up and giving thanks to God for the game I'm playing in that moment, the song I'm listening to, or whatever other activity I'm partaking in. I mean, how cool is it that He created these resources and gifted them to me?

Though I was absolutely shocked to learn this, God *wants* us to have fun and enjoy His creation. In Ecclesiastes 8:15, we're told, "So I recommend having fun, because there is nothing better for people in this world than to eat, drink, and enjoy life. That way they will experience some happiness along with all the hard work God gives them under the sun." And again, in Ecclesiastes 9:7-8, we read, "So go ahead. Eat your food with joy, and drink your wine with a happy heart, for God approves of this! Wear fine clothes, with a splash of cologne!"

It's important to note that the author is not saying that we should sin or just do whatever we want and abuse grace. That would contradict Romans 6, as well as the whole nature of God's Spirit indwelling us. Rather, as a commentary on *The Bible Says* states:

> Solomon set out to discover if pleasure would provide meaning to life, but found it wanting. Pleasure is an insufficient foundation for life. But that doesn't mean it isn't good. Solomon *commended pleasure*, stating there is *nothing better*. Since life is *vanity, we should embrace pleasure. To eat, drink, and be merry* is the best we are going to get in this life. But we can only truly enjoy these pleasures through the lens of fearing God and trusting Him by faith.[6]

Here's an illustration I often use. Let's say a parent buys a gift for their kid (again with the legitimately loving parent idea). Maybe it's a new game or LEGO set. They know their kid's going to love it, and they're stoked to give it to them. The point of giving that gift in the first place is for them to, you know, actually use it and enjoy it—ideally, for more than ten minutes. The good parent isn't going to give it to them and then turn around and say, "How dare you waste time with that meaningless thing! What's the matter with you?"

Likewise, how sad (and ungrateful) would it be if the kid threw it away upon receiving it? "No, this thing is worthless and I don't need it! Get it away from me! It won't make me productive, so I can't accept it."

Why do we think we have to do that with God's gifts? Why do we so often act like productivity is the sole purpose of every good thing? Just imagine that for a second. "Happy birthday, son! I got you a lawnmower and a toilet plunger. So, uh . . . get to it."

I'm not a parent and have no desire to be one, but I can at least deduce that such a scenario would be twisted.

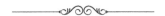

After years of playing a game of Musical Mentors, never quite clicking with any of them in that context, I got connected with Verity—the mentor who changed my life. She was the first Christian to understand my atypical brain and tell me I'm okay. This incredible woman with sage-level wisdom went on to help me work through my long list of anxieties, fighting my shame with me. It's crazy how legitimately scary it can feel to try to abandon negative and shameful thoughts about ourselves. I often feel that I'm not allowed to and that mentally abusing myself is the safest and most humble option. It's all a work in progress, but I'm in a much better place now.

I used to always call my intense daydreaming an addiction that I could never break no matter how hard I tried or how much I begged God to take it away or help me turn it off. Trying to stop felt like trying to grow taller or trying to will my eyes into turning blue. I felt completely alone in it, as I never met anyone who struggles with it like me—or who would admit it, anyway.

People frequently looked at me like I had three heads whenever I discussed it, which made me conclude for a long time that I was not only in sin but was also in weird, oddball, embarrassing sin that no one else on the planet wrestled with. Obviously, that's not the case. In fact, depending on one's heart, it's not even a sin. Verity was the first person to tell me that. Though I fought it hard at first, thinking the idea was completely outrageous, the burden that eventually left me was indescribable.

Throughout this journey these past few years—thanks, in large part, to Verity—I've accepted that my brain just ticks differently. I'm not neurotypical. My life and thought processes are going to contrast with most others. My daydreaming wasn't necessarily an addiction like I'd thought; it's just how my head is engineered. It's a core part of who I am. God gave me a creative mind.

Believe me, I'm not saying all of this just to make myself feel better or forcibly try to justify this thing. It's actually been kind of terrifying. I argued a lot with Verity when she told me it's actually okay for Christians to daydream and hyperfixate—something I never could've conceived of. This led to the most intense cognitive dissonance I've ever experienced.

"But it's idolatry!" I protested during one of our meetings. "It's evil, and I need to stop! Must destroy it at all costs!"

"Is it, though? Are you putting your faith in it to save you? Are you looking to it for salvation?"

"No, of course not."

"Then it's not an idol. You're not depending on it. You're just enjoying it and using your creative mind. Enjoying something a lot doesn't necessarily make it an idol, despite what many Christians like to say. Things have the potential to become idols. But everything you've ever said to me indicates that your primary concern is your relationship with God, and you want to love Him better."

"No, no, no. Listen to me. I'm a bad person. I am the filthiest of the filth because I daydream a lot, and it's *weird*."

"No, you're not. You're just a daydreamer, and you're allowed to be."

"But what if I'm not? What if I go to Hell because I failed to repent?"

"That will never happen. You are covered by the blood of Jesus."

"But—"

My anxiety monster still torments me over this, screaming questions in the back of my mind like, "What if I'm wrong? What if I'm just letting myself off the hook when I really should be trying to burn and destroy this thing? What if I'm the exception to forgiveness?" What if, what if, what if. And I imagine I'll probably have some level of anxiety over it for the rest of my life, unless I get a clear, Divine revelation with a completely straightforward answer. But either way, God is gracious. Jesus has me covered. We're only human, and none of us will get everything right in this life. There's no command for us to be completely, flawlessly correct in all of our theology in every area. That would be terrifying, and none of us would make it. We just ought to seek Him as best as we know how and be willing to receive and follow His guidance when we get it.

I always joke that there will be a frequently asked questions board in Heaven. One way or another, we'll all realize how wrong we were about so many things. I imagine we'll have a good laugh about it.

I later discussed the matter with some other people, including fellow neurodivergents, and that was even more encouraging. Second, third, fourth opinions are always helpful. Where does it state in Scripture that enjoying something a lot is idolatry? That was the big question. When the Israelites worshipped their statues, it wasn't the act of sculpting in itself that was the problem. They were looking to them for power and salvation instead of God. I don't think many of us look to our daydreams or our favorite shows as a means to salvation or view them as the ultimate source of life's meaning. We simply enjoy them—or hyperfixate in the case of neurodivergence. It's what our brains do.

Here's the idol test I give myself: if whatever special interest in question were to magically disappear from existence, devastating as that would be, how would I respond? Without God, I'd completely fall apart and would probably never recover (Exhibit A: what almost happened with the Melanie situation). But because He is faithful and far better than anything in this life, I know I'd be fine in the end. I'd mourn the loss, but life would still be worth living. I wouldn't be losing power, salvation, or any kind of ultimate satisfaction because only God can provide those things.

It's easy to repeat Christian clichés and popular ideas that we hear all the time in church. But how often do we pause and ask what they actually mean or what the specific implications are? What are examples of what they look like in everyday life beyond the obvious (don't murder; don't sleep around;

don't steal; don't forget to pray and read your Bible)? If these things are left vague, we can fall into the trap of assuming that anything and everything is bad. I think a prime example is how the term "idolatry" is thrown around like it applies to everything, always. We lose sight of what it actually means according to Scripture.

The group agreed that if someone thinks, "You like this thing way more than what *I* consider to be normal," it's just their opinion. Leave it as such. And regardless, shame is a terrible motivator. It makes me want to hide from God instead of running to Him. It's not just me, is it?

To clarify, when I previously said that I couldn't pray away my daydreaming, I'm not implying that we should always follow our feelings or assume God is cool with sin if the struggle doesn't disappear when we pray. That kind of thinking can become dangerous. But on this topic specifically, Scripture does not say that different neurotypes are evil. Scripture does not condemn having imaginations and putting them to use. Scripture does not say that we're not allowed to have hobbies outside of specific churchy things and enjoy them, even for lengthy periods of time.

I'm reminded of this quote from Ryan Ries in *Kill the Noise*: "You don't have to be one of those uptight, judgmental Christians who think that everything that's not cranked out by the church factory is evil. Just because a song isn't written by a well-known Christian artist doesn't mean that it's of the devil."[7]

As Jesus once said, "'It's not what goes into your mouth that defiles you; you are defiled by the words that come out of your mouth'" (Matt. 15:11). I think this applies to more than just literal food.

An important note regarding special interests: we need to be very careful in making sure that such intense hyperfixation isn't on real people in our lives, especially when it's unwelcome. Take what happened with Melanie and me as an example of how harmful that can be for both parties involved. When I discuss special interests, I'm referring to topics, activities, or pieces of media—those kinds of things.

Anime and video games, among other things, aren't Christian-based. But they're some of my favorite things, and I'm learning to allow myself to enjoy them. They've also paved the way for many wonderful friendships. I find a lot of value in exploring myself and the world through story and art, which can be done through creation and the imagination that God instills in people to put out their inspired content. God's Truth is reflected in all things, even if a piece of art or media wasn't specifically intended to have Christian themes. His glory and radiance shine through everything because we can't get away from Him, and it's awesome. As a famous Psalm says, "I can never escape from your Spirit! I can never get away from your presence! If I go up to heaven, you are there; if I go down to the grave, you are there. If I ride the wings of the morning, if I dwell by the farthest oceans, even there your hand will guide me, and your strength will support me" (Psalm 139:7-10).

There are so many awesome things out there to get a sense of wonder from and give God thanks for. For instance, playing the original *Spyro the Dragon* trilogy—my lifelong comfort games—*always* drives me to praise God. I'm reminded of some of the positive times in childhood and recognize God's kindness to me back then when I couldn't see it. When I watch *Naruto*, I'm struck by the beautifully artistic depictions of love, forgiveness, and repentance. When I recently strolled through the trails of Minoh Falls in Japan, I couldn't stop saying, "Man, God is so cool!" to myself amidst all the breathtaking scenery. I get similar feelings and a drive to worship when I listen to heavy rock music. When I cuddle with an adorable cat, I get a heart-warming, faded reflection of God's affectionate love and adoration. To claim that church, singing, and Bible reading are the only ways to experience God is to limit and dishonor God.

"But Miya," I hear you say, "we shouldn't be indulging in worldly things!"

Okay, I hear you. But what are worldly things, exactly? Anything that isn't specifically Christian-brand? The Bible specifically refers to worldly things as greed, sexual immorality, rage, slander, lying, etc. (Col. 3:5-9). Not conforming to this world means not shamelessly living in sin with no reverence for God like those who have rejected Him. Instead, we are to have "tenderhearted mercy, kindness, humility, gentleness, and patience" (Col. 3:12).

There will always be individuals who advise against engaging in "meaningless" activities, promoting unreasonable self-denial, and prioritizing solely "spiritual" matters. I hear heartbreaking stories about this from other Christians all the time. But as I would be astonished to discover, Paul actually speaks *against* asceticism, or extreme self-denial. There will always be Christians trying to disqualify others from the faith. Paul speaks against that, too.

> So don't let anyone condemn you for what you eat or drink, or for not celebrating certain holy days or new moon ceremonies or Sabbaths. For these rules are only shadows of the reality yet to come. And Christ himself is that reality. Don't let anyone condemn you by insisting on pious self-denial or the worship of angels, saying they have had visions about these things. Their sinful minds have made them proud, and they are not connected to Christ, the head of the body. For he holds the whole body together with its joints and ligaments, and it grows as God nourishes it.
>
> You have died with Christ, and he has set you free from the spiritual powers of this world. So why do you keep on following the rules of the world, such as, "Don't handle! Don't taste! Don't touch!"? Such rules are mere human teachings about things that deteriorate as we use them. These rules may seem wise because they require strong devotion, pious self-denial, and severe bodily discipline. But they provide no help in conquering a person's evil desires (Col. 2:18-23).

In short, Jesus is enough, guys. Quit adding extra stuff. It's not about legalism.

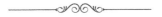

I think there are plenty of other Christians out there who feel as though they struggle with things like daydreaming and fantasy. Many think it's this horrible, embarrassing thing like I did for so long—especially if one's fixation is on something considered childish (which is usually subjective and debatable). It shouldn't be that way. If the thing in question isn't inherently sinful and isn't causing the person to stumble, I believe it should be enjoyed without being a source of guilt. This should be something we all feel safe talking about, recognizing that it isn't shameful and doesn't make us bad Christians.

But that's the thing. No one ever talks about it. It makes us feel alone in our struggles or what causes us to believe they're immoral things to struggle with in the first place. The silence creates an illusion that these things don't exist and don't happen to anyone else. For instance, I've never heard of a support group for maladaptive daydreaming. It's not the norm for Bible study leaders to write lessons on neurodiversity and special interests (and in a positive, affirming manner). These types of conversations tend to exist solely in niche internet spaces.

To be clear, I do think there can come a point where daydreaming and fixations can become so severe that they heavily and negatively affect one's daily life or cause a neglect of responsibilities, and getting professional help is a good way to go. But I'm not a mental health expert, so I can't really go into depth on that or offer advice. All I can say is, Christians, whatever our special thing is, it's good to remember that one of the fruits of the Spirit is self-control. Sometimes, when I've been really invested in something, I need to take a step back and chill out for a bit, like the times when I'd play and replay the *Persona* series back-to-back, stacking up hundreds of hours and leaving very little time or brain space for other things. That doesn't necessarily mean I have to stop forever. It means giving it a rest and not letting it completely take over my life. Personal limits and balances can vary from one person to the next.

Whether it's daydreaming, fandom, or whatever thing we feel ashamed about, I think it's helpful and even dignified (yes, really) to speak up about it, even if it feels weird or unusual. It took me twenty-two years to finally open up to trusted friends about my baggage and unconventional struggles after much conviction. I think if it becomes more of a normal conversation, a lot of us will find that maybe it's not so shameful after all. Maybe it's a lot more common than we think. You never know who might be listening, waiting for that one person to take the lead before they feel brave enough to share their own story.

# CHAPTER SEVENTEEN
## We Are Valid

There's a particular level of heartache that's evoked when I hear neurodivergent Christians say they don't feel welcome in church settings because of their differences. I'm lucky to be a member of a good church where I'm accepted even while being openly autistic. Sadly, that seems to be more on the unusual side, based on what I hear from others.

Let's talk about a piece of Christian media that's actually phenomenal and not cheesy. In the TV series *The Chosen,* the disciple Matthew is heavily autistic-coded in his portrayal. While that's merely a speculation and not biblically canon concerning the real Matthew and while I'm always wary of autism representation in the media (especially when it's centered around stereotypes), I deeply appreciate this. It reminds me in a unique way that Jesus loves autistic people and wants autistic followers.

Jesus doesn't heal Matthew's autism. It's not even brought up as an issue. As with all His disciples, Jesus is concerned about the heart, not about whether Matthew can perfectly comply with social and cultural standards.

For a while, many of the other disciples didn't accept him due to his background as a tax collector. When I watch it, however, I empathize for a different reason. The way he's mistreated for his social struggles could be looked at as a standalone thing, regardless of his former profession. A scene that stuck out to me was when he had a question about Scripture but tells Mary Magdalene that he'd rather talk to Philip than the others because Philip is nice to him. Saddened, Mary apologizes that he's been the exception. Regardless, Matthew is set on taking the question to someone he feels safe with—away from the rest of the group where he regularly feels hated and unwanted.[8]

I'll admit, there aren't a whole lot of hills in life that I'd want to die on. But one exception is my belief that people should be allowed to show up as themselves in God's family. In a world where we constantly have to mask to get by, a community of fellow believers of all places should be a safe space to stop faking it and be real. Church shouldn't be a fake or insincere place.

We should be allowed to take off the mask and be as delightfully awkward as we naturally are, without being put down or isolated for it. We should be allowed to discuss our differences and challenges without fear of being told that our neurology is from the devil and needs to be cast out. We should be allowed to harmlessly stim without fearing punishment or reprimand. (Stimming is a soothing, self-regulating response to different emotions and stimuli, such as rocking, leg shaking, rapid blinking, hand flapping, hair twirling, etc. Neurotypicals stim, too, but usually much less frequently.) If I had a dollar for every time I wasn't able to pay attention to what someone was saying because I was so focused on trying not to do my eye stims, I'd have a lot of dollars.

Even though *The Chosen* is, as I like to say, kind of like fanfiction in certain areas, I just think it would be really cool if neurodivergent people could be seen and treated with dignity and kindness like that of Phillip, Thaddeus, and Jesus toward Matthew.

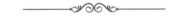

For the longest time, I thought it was only okay to talk about the bad stuff if it was past tense, especially in church settings. I spent nearly a decade claiming that I *used to* be a depressed and solitary individual and that I *once* was autistic but no longer. (This one is a big oof. I apologize profusely on behalf of my past self.)

Obviously, autism never went away, though I genuinely believed it did for a long time, as discussed earlier. Being autistic isn't a bad thing, so

I shouldn't have been trying to flex about "conquering" it in the first place. As for the other stuff, depression comes and goes. For most of us, it's not something that gets overcome one time and then it's gone forever. I had to learn that just because I'm not bubbly and talkative all the time doesn't mean I'm an unfriendly person or a bad Christian. Not being perpetually cheerful doesn't mean I'm not living in victory. I'm not biblically commanded to be Buddy the Elf every waking moment. And, of course, being a quiet loner isn't necessarily bad either. Though underappreciated, there's immense value in thoughtful, quiet strength. I'm certainly a lot more mindful and considerate now than I was back when the entirety of my brain energy was spent on being a chatterbox at all costs.

Despite the fear of being judged, I've come to learn this wild idea that I can talk about present tense struggles, too—including ways that I actively sin in the present. While doing so isn't as popular as sharing victory stories, it's dangerously prideful and utterly foolish to act as if all my sins are in the past and that I do no wrong anymore. As James 5:16 says, "Confess your sins to each other and pray for each other so that you may be healed. The earnest prayer of a righteous person has great power and produces wonderful results."

Around the time when I began to wonder if I was "still" autistic, my soon-to-be mentor Verity had gone up on stage at church and explained that she was interested in mentoring fellow neurodivergent people and trying to find ways together of growing and getting closer with God and each other outside of just the usual traditional methods. It sounded like a good match.

Our first meetup was scheduled after I sent an anxious essay of a text on why I thought I might not make it to Heaven. I was ready. It was time to list out all the reasons why I was the worst human alive and ask for a magical solution about how to repent of my weirdness.

We arrived at the outdoor café and I unloaded all of my garbage, assuming that the sinful nature of it all, especially daydreaming, was a given.

"*Obviously,* this stuff is all terrible and abominable to God, so tell me how to stop doing it."

"But I don't see how that's a sin at all. Who told you that?"

Utterly flabbergasted, I listened as the first person in the two-and-a-half decades I'd been alive told me I was not sinning by being myself, that daydreaming isn't evil or shameful, and that I don't have to imprison myself.

My eventual diagnosis further verified that I was fine.

"You're autistic," Verity said afterward. "It makes perfect sense that you have intense special interests."

Since then, though it's been an ongoing journey, I've experienced an abundance of freedom, despite the challenges. Christ has set me free, after all.

I might not have gone up that day if I wasn't willing to admit or even acknowledge my own neurodivergence, even if it was just a hunch at the time. Being honest about it has allowed me to meet and connect with people similar to me, and it's been life-changing.

Don't get me wrong—I'm not someone who believes that autism is a superpower, and it certainly doesn't make us *better* than neurotypical people. But it's not a disease either. It's not a bad word. It's just a thing—a thing that's different and so often misunderstood.

There are struggles, and it's important to acknowledge them. At the same time, it's good to appreciate the positives, like how in many ways, we get to have a magnified sense of wonder for God and His creation. We are not invalid. We are not less-than. We are loved by God just as much as any allistic person.

As a disclaimer, when I say that we are valid, that is not to say that we are perfect. It's not to say that we should love every single thing about ourselves. As humans, we all sin all the time. It's important to remember that we're not supposed to love our sin, regardless of the reasoning for it. We are called to have repentant hearts and place our faith in Jesus to save us, as it's literally impossible to do so ourselves. Autistic or not, we all need a Savior.

Keeping that in mind, being autistic does not take away any of our value as God's created masterpieces. With church culture often expressing disapproval toward things that I've discussed, such as loving fiction and fantasy to socially abnormal levels, I spent many years thinking I needed to literally repent of my brain—repent of being autistic. That's not a thing.

It all goes back to the question, what does the Bible classify as sin, and what is just human judgment and assumptions? What is biblically accurate, and what is just cultural Christianity? Just because an idea is repeated continually over a period of time doesn't necessarily mean it's biblically correct. For example, many people to this day still think the saying, "God helps those who help themselves," is a Bible verse. It's not.

Context in the Bible is everything. Sometimes we look at individual verses, and sometimes we look at the big picture. I've heard countless well-meaning preachers and influencers say that things like games, videos, manga, and so on are all wastes of time and that we need to be living for Jesus instead. As discussed earlier, I strongly believe that these things don't have to be mutually exclusive. What many neurodivergent people hear in these kinds of messages—those whose special interests are games, videos, manga, and so on—is: "Your passions and interests are stupid, and you're living in sin. You're not allowed to do those things anymore because they're pointless. Throw them all away."

Due largely to the lack of real autism awareness and understanding in the world, a lot of said preachers and influencers don't think about that. I don't think they realize that these things they see as meaningless are actually ways that many people uniquely connect with God and worship Him. As neurodiversity becomes more of a conversation with less stigma, I think it would be helpful for us all to be mindful of these things. (And of course, this doesn't apply only to neurodiversity. Neurotypicals can enjoy things intensely, too).

It's like Daniel Bowman Jr. says in his excellent book *On the Spectrum*: "In my case, my autistic brain wiring leads me to see storytelling and poetry and teaching and learning and worshiping God in ways that are different from what most readers will be accustomed to. I hope you're open to exploring those new ways alongside me, wherever they lead."[9]

Different people's walks with God don't have to look identical. Living for Jesus and enjoying our interests don't have to be separate things. First Corinthians 10:31 says, "So whether you eat or drink, or whatever you do, do it all for the glory of God." I used to interpret that as, "Literally everything you do, including eating, has to be Jesus-brand. You have to hold your breath, strain yourself, and make sure your brain is super-duper focused on God every second no matter what you're doing." After being gently and lovingly challenged in that way of thinking, I now read that verse differently. *Whatever* you do can include "non-spiritual" things as well. All of life is for Jesus. We can do anything, even simple and basic things like eating and drinking, all to the glory of God. The ways we can glorify Him are too many to count.

Another of my favorites, *Aggressively Happy* by Joy Marie Clarkson, backs this up beautifully.

> Scripture says to "love the Lord your God with all your heart and with all your soul and with all your mind and with all your strength" (Mark 12:30). It is easy to spiritualize this verse, as though we only love God with our minds by thinking about God. But I like to think that living into the fullness of our capacities in each of these areas is loving God. It is not merely about the content of our loving, but the preposition; we do these things with God. When we use our minds to ponder the complexities of quantum entanglement, we are loving God with our minds. When we run a marathon, or reach the top of our class, or salsa dance, we are loving God with our strength. When we love someone with our whole heart or pour all that we are into a cause that matters, we are loving God with our soul. Let's not give God less credit than God deserves. If God created us with

the capacity to be interesting, skilled, intelligent, and cultured, why do we assume God only desires placid little devotees who read only Bible study books and eat only oatmeal?[10]

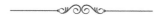

Don't worry—I know I can't end a discussion like this without addressing the Great Commission. Get ready for a ramble, and remember that these are my non-universal views.

I believe that autistic people have unique voices (whether that's a physical voice or communicating through other methods—all are completely valid) and that autistic Christians can be missional in unique ways. Maybe that means having spiritual conversations with people we met through special interests, whether online or otherwise. Maybe it means creating fanfiction, fanart, or original content that reflects Christ and the gospel. Maybe it means connecting with people at church who are overwhelmed by big crowds. Maybe it's writing our stories. Maybe it's educating people about autism and how to better love autistic people. Maybe it's not doing anything flashy but praying and worshiping God in one's own ways that are just as valid. There are all kinds of possibilities. We're called to be missional as followers of Christ, but it doesn't always have to look the same for everyone.

This doesn't have to translate to "you must evangelize at all times." I'm still unlearning that one. Simply being a friend to people, showing kindness, making art, enjoying God's creation and gifts, and being the sort of people He made us to be are all glorifying to Him. Evangelism is certainly a gift some people have (Eph. 4:11), and many folks have that calling. I don't think any of us should intentionally shirk opportunities that come our way. But overall, I've come to believe that we don't need to live with the pressure of feeling like we have to preach at everyone we meet. In this day and age, that seems to be an almost surefire way to turn someone off, unless doing so actually makes sense in a specific situation. I'd imagine most of us don't want to be perceived as "a noisy gong or a clanging cymbal" (1 Cor. 13:1). Discussions are good but they shouldn't be forced or manipulated. It's usually helpful to have a relationship with the person first, but we shouldn't deceptively befriend people with hidden agendas. There are ways to make disciples—not as car salesmen but by showing Who Jesus is through our lives and the fruit we bear. "But the Holy Spirit produces this kind of fruit in our lives: love, joy, peace, patience, kindness, goodness, faithfulness, gentleness, and self-control. There is no law against these things!" (Gal. 5:22-23).

I don't think we have to force everything to be super obviously spiritual, unless perhaps one feels specifically convicted by God to do so (actual conviction, not anxiety). When I look back at some of my old creations that I forced clear, in-your-face Christianity into out of obligation, trying to earn my right to create art at all, it was very over-the-top and very cringey. That's not to say that making Christian art isn't a wonderful thing—as long as that's actually what someone is feeling led to do and it's not an internalized guilt trip or forced obligation.

We can have a relationship with God in a way that feels natural to us. It doesn't always have to look exactly like what fancy theology books tell us about how to be a "good" Christian. I, for one, have grown exhausted from the shame that comes from not being able to meet many of those standards consistently. No one needs to carry that shame around. Even those ideal "good Christian" lifestyles can become idols. We can fall into the trap of believing that works and respectable behaviors are what save us.

I try to keep in mind the fact that most sermons and theology books aren't written for a neurodivergent audience. A lot of things they tell us we're supposed to do as Christians aren't always feasible for everyone. And that's okay. We do what we can. In the end, God wants our hearts, not an impressive résumé.

Neurodivergent people are so valuable to God's Kingdom. Diversity is a beautiful thing. Not everyone can be an eye, or a hand, or a foot (Rom. 12:4-8). But we are all important parts of the body of Christ. It wouldn't exactly be a body if it was just a bunch of eyeballs. If I'm just a fingernail, then I'm happy to become the best fingernail I can be. I mean, I think I at least do a somewhat decent job of scratching away at the old, crusty paint layer of lies and stereotypes surrounding both autism and Christianity, even if it's just a small corner of the wall. And there are other fingernails out there helping to do the same. God can use us in miraculous ways, even when we feel completely inadequate and even if those ways aren't flashy. An old pastor of mine would often quote the famous line, "God doesn't call the equipped—He equips the called."

# CHAPTER EIGHTEEN
## God Adores My Quirky Brain

If I'm honest, I felt completely unqualified to write a book. I'm not an expert on anything, I'm probably a mediocre writer at best, and I've never even been a huge reader. Someone like me shouldn't be allowed to write a real book. In other words, imposter syndrome has never wanted to be my friend so badly.

I was on a drive home with my husband from Bible study one night, exhausted and destroyed in every possible way, feeling hopeless in ever figuring out what I actually wanted to do with my life. After some silence, he suddenly asked, "Have you ever thought about writing a book?"

Yes, I had for a long time. But I forgot about it. I wanted to in college when Lacey Sturm's book *The Reason* came out and inspired me. I knew that was the kind of book I wanted to write if I ever dared to make an attempt, so I started the brainstorming process by word vomiting incoherent thoughts about my life. But then it occurred to me that only famous people get published. Becoming a legitimate author was next to impossible for a nobody like me, so I discarded the idea and never touched it again.

"I hardly even read books," I replied. "I'm not qualified to write one."

"You know, that actually seems to be a common thing. Most of the professional podcasters I listen to admit they don't listen to other podcasts. That doesn't have to be a reason to hold you back. I think a lot of people find it refreshing whenever you're vulnerable and talk about things that no one else ever talks about."

After that, I began thinking. God is bigger than my lack of qualifications. He is bigger than my insecurities. If I write a book and He wants to do something with it, I need to trust that He will.

I began working on this book the next day. And then my habit of never reading evolved to the point of needing to buy multiple bookshelves.

I've wanted to share my story with the world since that first time at church when I graduated high school. I want God to be magnified and His creation to be encouraged. Even if the book ends up flopping, I trust He will still be glorified somehow.

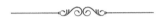

Confession: I can vent a lot sometimes, even when I'm literally not upset about a thing anymore. Maybe it's an autistic info-dump thing. I do enjoy doing that. I tried my best to not come off as a complainer in this book, even when describing painful events, though I guess that's up for interpretation. I truly have had a blessed life.

Even if I hadn't had all those struggles, was never disabled, was always killing it socially, and had been popular and looked up to by people, I still would've come away empty and unfulfilled in the end if I had never found God. King Solomon, probably the wisest man in history second to Jesus, writes from his own experience throughout Ecclesiastes about how you can obtain everything life has to offer and still find that it's all vanity in the end. It wouldn't have mattered if I had gotten everything I thought I wanted from the beginning. Only the Maker of my heart can ultimately fill the void inside of it.

I probably sound like a broken record at this point, but it's so important: God's love is unconditional. No matter what we do or what we've done, His love never changes. It's hard for me to fathom even now, especially since love from people is so conditional, always. Even though I logically know better, anxiety still gets the best of me now and then. I think a lot of it has to do with the toxic messages that many of us have gotten throughout our lives, even if indirectly.

"Yes, God's love is unconditional, and the cross is sufficient, *but* you still have to do X, Y, Z to *really* be saved."

I struggle to shake this mindset sometimes. The cursed anxiety monster and what I know to be true go to war in my head on a near-constant basis. It's probably a literal battlefield up there. People are slashing at each other with their weapons; soldiers are getting knocked out on both sides, even as they take cover; and maybe there's an occasional explosion or someone sets the scene on fire. Both sides think they're right, and once one side thinks it's winning, someone hiding in the distance shoots a bunch of their guys with arrows.

I've been trained to always focus more on defense than offense in order to survive those fatal blows. Much of this is thanks to my experience with so-called love from people, teaching me to always keep my guard up. All the times people changed their minds. All the "I love you, *but* . . . " comments and insinuations. All the people who tried to control me through threats and intimidation and called it love. All the pretending and deception. All the ticking bombs eagerly waiting for me to make a wrong move.

These things I've been conditioned to expect aren't reflective of our loving, merciful God. There are consequences for our actions in life, but God doesn't delight in our suffering. He doesn't look down on us with crossed arms and a disapproving glare as we come to Him. He also doesn't look at us with a smug, sadistic smirk and say, "Shame on you, idiot! What did I tell ya?"

When we come back to Him, He looks at us like the father of the prodigal son: weeping with joy and throwing a party in Heaven (Luke 15:11-32). He rejoices over His lost sheep returning home. We are made into royalty.

Note to self and anyone else who needs it: take a deep breath. You're going to be okay. Jesus has already won.

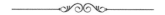

When it comes down to it, I'm just a person—a speck of dust—and I'm not that important in the grand scheme of things. But all the same, I am in the sense that I'm a cherished, irreplaceable child of God, whom He made intentionally as part of His narrative. None of us are the main character in the ultimate story. That role belongs to Jesus alone. What I couldn't see in my B.C. days was the mind-boggling fact that the world doesn't revolve around me.

Life isn't about my pain and desires. It's not about me trying to be well-liked (which is a hard pill to swallow even now). Some people will hate me for my faith, and some will never understand my neurodivergence. And that's okay. I am a whosoever. "'For God so loved the world, that he gave his only begotten Son, that *whosoever* believeth in him should not perish, but have everlasting life'" (John 3:16, KJV, emphasis mine). That may be the most well-known pillow verse, but it's so important. It helps me to remember my place.

Yes, I'm autistic. Yes, I also acknowledge the difficulties I face in life as a result in a broken society that isn't really designed for people like me. But even if I didn't face these challenges and felt like I was brilliantly adept at everything, it wouldn't matter. I'm still a whosoever made of dust.

I will say that it's encouraging to see that, at least in some ways, culture seems to be slowly drifting toward neurodiversity acceptance and understanding. Let's keep it going. Let's fight for a world where autistic people don't feel like they're only allowed to exist in internet spaces. Let's fight for a Church culture where neurodivergent individuals genuinely feel like they belong. Let's fight for a society that doesn't try to cram square pegs into round holes—one where we can tell people we've been diagnosed with autism and their automatic response isn't, "Oh no! I'm *so* sorry," but rather, "Congratulations! That's awesome that you made such an important discovery about yourself. Let's go out for ice cream and celebrate!"

Let's fight to end the stigma.

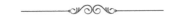

Sometimes I'm asked, "How could anyone even believe in God? Why is that still a thing?" And I never know how to answer in the moment.

My first instinct is to say, "It helps to have encounters with Him," though that sounds oversimplified and probably obnoxious, since it's not like we can exactly control that. But encounters can look very different for different people. It doesn't always have to be a crazy, magical moment. It doesn't even have to be emotional, necessarily. Maybe it's an unexpected Paul-like experience, or maybe it's through something like studying apologetics. People have all kinds of different stories of how they've experienced Jesus, and the diversity is something to behold. You hear testimonies from Lacey Sturm to David Wood to Brian Welch to Lee Strobel. A massively important aspect, however, is pursuing Him.

I'm not sure I would've truly believed if I had just browsed through a Bible one day with no real context or just looked at the state of the world and listened to culture. Maybe I would have, but I have my doubts. It would've been so easy to be swayed. Don't mind me as I timidly point back to the "community is important" piece from earlier.

Ultimately, all I can say when those kinds of questions come up is to seek God humbly, in your own way—assuming the person asking isn't trolling but is genuinely curious and desires to seek God on some level. My story didn't end with Him reaching out to me that one day, and then everything was magical ever since. I had to work at our relationship and pursue Him continually. Otherwise, that day would've just been a nice moment, but once the high wore off, I would've gone back to the way I was before. My heart needed to be willing. I needed to humble myself and be eager to grow.

Jeremiah 29:13-14 says, "'If you look for me wholeheartedly, you will find me. I will be found by you,' says the Lord." Something I notice in this passage is that it doesn't say, "You will find me *immediately*." It doesn't say, "Seek me, and then I'll get back to you in three to five business days." For some people, it may happen quickly. For others, it can take a long time. I implore anyone who's on this journey and it seems like nothing's happening to not lose heart. Keep going.

I personally didn't need to know a bunch of deep theology or hear compelling arguments in order to be reached by God and want to pursue Him. It's not always about that. I didn't go to church or read the Bible until later on. It started with prayer and surrender. It started with a genuine desire for a relationship. And just like with any relationship, it's not just based on emotions. We won't have the feels all the time. It's an intentional, committed choice—one that we continue to make throughout our lifetimes.

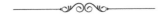

I know a lot of what I've said is bound to be met with disagreement. I anticipate pushback for challenging Church culture norms and presenting ideas that aren't popular or trendy. I won't even be surprised if I get comments like, "If you're not an expert with a bunch of degrees in mental health, autism, theology, or any other topic, then you don't have the right to talk about them!"

But none of that changes the fact that this is my story. I'm not an expert theologian and probably never will be. I'm going to get things wrong. It's part of being human. "Now we see things imperfectly, like puzzling reflections in a mirror," Paul says, "but then we will see everything with perfect clarity. All that I know now is partial and incomplete, but then I will know everything completely, just as God now knows me completely" (1 Cor. 13:12).

My primary purpose is to encourage, not to argue or be an automated apologetics machine for random interrogations. My autistic brain tends to process things more slowly in general, so I'd probably make for a lousy debater, anyway.

Civil conversations are different from interrogations and attacks. I'm much more open to a good, respectful discussion with a friend, where we can ask questions, listen, and try to understand one another better. But again, I don't have all the answers and wouldn't dare pretend otherwise. I'm just a regular layperson trying her best.

That's where most of us are. I don't think we should feel as though we don't have a voice and aren't allowed to share our thoughts just because we're not professional scholars. Although I'm not a fan of how my voice sounds, God still gave me a voice and the privilege of using it. I want to use it in all of its forms to bring glory to Him and encouragement to others as best as my imperfect self can. I might not be great at it, but God still sees my heart. "For when I am weak, then I am strong" (2 Cor. 12:10).

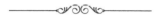

There's lots of cool stuff growing in the garden. Lots of carrots. Lots of radishes. Lots of cucumbers. And one awkward potato. The other vegetables wondered why the potato didn't look like them. They looked down on the potato. They excluded the potato from their fun veggie hangouts.

But this awkward potato now knows where her value comes from and that she is valid being the potato she was created to be. She doesn't have to transform into a carrot, radish, or cucumber. Her worth was never meant to lie in the opinions of man. Or plants.

"Thank you for making me so wonderfully complex! Your workmanship is marvelous—how well I know it" (Psalm 139:14). Cheers to embracing life as the distinctive individuals we were each created to be.

# About the Author

Miya Sae was diagnosed with autism at age twenty-six. She gave her life to God after a miraculous encounter and has been actively pursuing Him ever since. Miya is a graduate of Northern Arizona University with a degree in social work. She is continually learning how to navigate the world as a neurodivergent Christian in a joyful manner and aspires to help others do the same.

Forever a Pokémon master at heart, Miya loves to dream, write, explore ideas, and occasionally make amateur-level fanart. When not creating content, she's usually watching anime, gaming, or petting her cats until they get annoyed. She currently lives in Arizona with her husband and their two felines, Nebby and Mochi.

# Endnotes

1 Sara Gibbs, Drama Queen: One Autistic Woman and a Life of Unhelpful Labels (London: Headline, 2021), 6.

2 Brant Hansen, Blessed Are the Misfits: Great News For Believers Who Are Introverts, Spiritual Strugglers, Or Just Feel Like They're Missing Something (Nashville: Thomas Nelson, 2017), 100.

3 Dane Ortlund, Gently and Lowly: The Heart of Christ for Sinners and Sufferers (Wheaton: Crossway, 2020), 30.

4 Susan Cain, Quiet: The Power of Introverts in a World That Can't Stop Talking (New York: Crown, 2012), 6.

5 Jim Sinclair, "Don't Mourn for Us," Our Voice, 1, No. 3 (1993): 1-2. https://doi.org/10.1007/978-981-13-8437-0_2.

6 "Ecclesiastes 8:14-15 Meaning," The Bible Says online, accessed November 2, 2022, https://thebiblesays.com/commentary/eccl/eccl-8/ecclesiastes-814-15/.

7 Ryan Ries, Kill the Noise: Finding Meaning Above the Madness (New York: FaithWords, 2021), 81.

8 The Chosen, Season 2, Episode 2, "I Saw You," directed by Dallas Jenkins, Aired April 13, 2021, on Angel Studios, https://www.angel.com/watch/the-chosen/episode/d4a7ed5d-2805-4879-90e7-c906a6fabea8/season-2/episode-2/i-saw-you184683594354.

9 Daniel Bowman Jr., On the Spectrum: Autism, Faith, & the Gifts of Neurodiversity (Grand Rapids: Brazos Press, 2021), 38.

10 Joy Marie Clarkson, Aggressively Happy: A Realist's Guide to Believing in the Goodness of Life (Bloomington: Bethany House Publishers, 2022), 56-57.

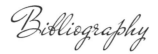

# Bibliography

Bowman, Jr., Daniel. *On the Spectrum: Autism, Faith, & the Gifts of Neurodiversity.* Grand Rapids: Brazos Press, 2021.

Cain, Susan. *Quiet: The Power of Introverts in a World That Can't Stop Talking.* New York: Crown, 2012.

*Chosen, The.* Season 2. Episode 2. "I Saw You." Directed by Dallas Jenkins. Aired April 13, 2021, on Angel Studios. https://www.angel.com/watch/the-chosen/episode/d4a7ed5d-2805-4879-90e7-c906a6fabea8/season-2/episode-2/i-saw-you184683594354.

Clarkson, Joy Marie. *Aggressively Happy: A Realist's Guide to Believing in the Goodness of Life.* Bloomington: Bethany House Publishers, 2022.

"Ecclesiastes 8:14-15 Meaning." The Bible Says online. Accessed November 2, 2022. https://thebiblesays.com/commentary/eccl/eccl-8/ecclesiastes-814-15/.

Gibbs, Sara. *Drama Queen: One Autistic Woman and a Life of Unhelpful Labels.* London: Headline, 2021.

Hansen, Brant. *Blessed Are the Misfits: Great News For Believers Who Are Introverts, Spiritual Strugglers, Or Just Feel Like They're Missing Something.* Nashville: Thomas Nelson, 2017.

Ortlund, Dane. *Gently and Lowly: The Heart of Christ for Sinners and Sufferers.* Wheaton: Crossway, 2020.

Ries, Ryan. *Kill the Noise: Finding Meaning Above the Madness.* New York: FaithWords, 2021.

Sinclair, Jim. "Don't Mourn for Us." *Our Voice.* 1. No. 3 (1993): 1-2. https://doi.org/10.1007/978-981-13-8437-0_2.

Ambassador International's mission is to magnify the Lord Jesus Christ and promote His Gospel through the written word.

We believe through the publication of Christian literature, Jesus Christ and His Word will be exalted, believers will be strengthened in their walk with Him, and the lost will be directed to Jesus Christ as the only way of salvation.

## For more information about
## AMBASSADOR INTERNATIONAL
## please visit:

*www.ambassador-international.com*
*@AmbassadorIntl*
*www.facebook.com/AmbassadorIntl*

*Thank you for reading this book!*

*You make it possible for us to fulfill our mission, and we are grateful for your partnership.*

*To help further our mission, please consider leaving us a review on your social media, favorite retailer's website, Goodreads or Bookbub, or our website, and check out some of the books on the following page!*

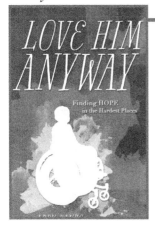

One night can change everything. Abby Banks put her healthy, happy infant son to sleep, but when she awoke the next morning, she felt as though she was living a nightmare. Her son, Wyatt, was paralyzed. In an instant, all her hopes and dreams for him were wiped away. As she struggled to come to grips with her son's devastating diagnosis and difficult rehabilitation, she found true hope in making a simple choice, a choice to love anyway—to love her son, the life she didn't plan, and the God of hope, Who is faithful even when the healing doesn't come.

Are you dealing with chronic illness? Do you ever feel like you're on this journey alone, that no one else understands you? Well, you are not alone. In this journal of dealing with chronic illness, Daphne Self is raw and open about her own struggles with an invisible disease and with the God Who created her and allows suffering for now. Follow Daphne's thirty entries of how she deals with her own disabilities and how she finds comfort and peace in the arms of her Savior.

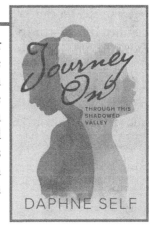

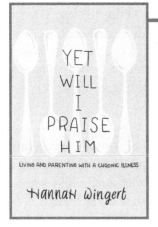

After being diagnosed with a chronic illness, Hannah Wingert has had to come to terms with her diagnosis and to learn to be a wife and mother in the midst of her invisible illness. In *Yet Will I Praise Him*, Hannah opens up candidly about her own struggles of living and parenting with a chronic illness. She will help you understand how to use your chronic illness to grow in your faith, how to balance your marriage and parenting, and how to live each day with hope so you can not only survive the challenges you face, but also thrive.

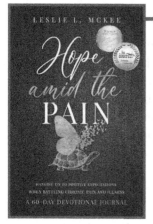

Millions of women suffering from chronic pain and illness want the reassurance they're not alone. The devotions in *Hope Amid the Pain* are written by a chronic pain warrior with over twenty-five years' experience and will point the reader to hope and encouragement. It's possible to Hang On to Positive Expectations (HOPE) even amid the pain."

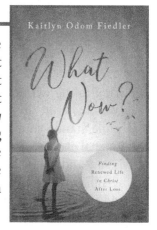

Kaitlyn Odom Fiedler was eight years old when she became the victim of a horrible car accident that claimed the lives of six of her family members. Left with only one living brother, young Kaitlyn was left with the question, "What now?" *What Now?: Finding Renewed Life in Christ After Loss* brings a refreshing perspective of hope and will help answer the questions of how to move forward, not just move on, when it seems there is nothing left on which to cling.

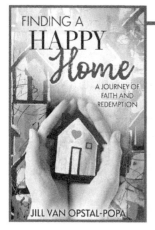

Growing up in small-town Ohio, Jill van Opstal-Popa never dreamed she would be making her home among the orphaned children of Brazil. But when she and her husband set out to be missionaries, they found themselves building a home for the children who had no home.

In *Finding a Happy Home: A Journey of Faith and Redemption,* from the heart of a mother to many comes the stories of the people of Brazil. Your heart will be pulled to the stories of each child whose story is unique but also like so many others.

Made in the USA
Middletown, DE
23 April 2025

74654927R00116